Ectopic Pregnancy

Get the support you need, recover effectively and boost your fertility for future pregnancy

Including guide to symptoms, causes, treatment and recovery

By Claudia Gordon

CONTENTS

Foreword

If you're reading this book, then chances are you've been diagnosed with an ectopic pregnancy or you know someone who has. The diagnosis of an ectopic pregnancy is generally a surprise. In fact, some women didn't even realize they were pregnant at all and were experiencing mild symptoms, such as abdominal pain and tenderness or spotting, that they attributed to something else. Others might have had a positive pregnancy test and assumed the symptoms were the normal signs of early pregnancy. As a result, the diagnosis of an ectopic pregnancy usually comes as a shock and can be very painful and traumatic.

Today, ectopic pregnancies account for 1-2% of all conceptions. An ectopic pregnancy is considered an early embryo that implants outside of the uterus, usually in the fallopian tubes, although it can implant in other areas of the abdomen and pelvic region. It can be an extremely serious medical condition and even life-threatening but these days that risk is extremely low.

Thanks to modern technology and the use of early detection systems like transvaginal ultrasound most ectopic pregnancies are caught in the early stages of pregnancy and treated before they become very serious and cause damage to the fallopian tubes and other organs.

Although there is an increased risk of having multiple ectopic pregnancies, 60-65% of women who've experienced an ectopic pregnancy do go on to have a subsequent healthy pregnancy within 18 months.

Of course not everyone will want to try to conceive again. If you're one of the ones who does want to - the figure should be re-assuring as it obviously doesn't include either those who do go on to have a successful pregnancy *after* 18 months - and the remaining 35-40% includes those who are *not* trying to conceive again. Although you may feel devastated about your loss, and incredibly scared about a subsequent pregnancy, keep in mind that most people who want to try again *are* successful – and this book can help you ensure you're doing all you can to fully recover and prepare your body for future pregnancy.

In the following book, we'll go over what an ectopic pregnancy is, some of the common causes, the treatment options, what you can expect from the various treatments, and what the chances of recurrence truly mean.

If you want to try to conceive again we'll look at ways you can boost your fertility quickly to ensure you give yourself the best possible chance of success.

The diagnosis of an ectopic pregnancy can leave you feeling confused, scared, and helpless. This book aims to help you fight that fear with practical, relevant information, and empower you to take your health and life back under your control again.

Introduction

In the majority of ectopic pregnancies, the egg attaches to the fallopian tube, which is why sometimes ectopic pregnancies are referred to as "tubal pregnancies." Ectopic pregnancies are very serious. If they deteriorate, they can cause internal bleeding, infection, and even death in rare cases. Although mortality rates for ectopic pregnancies are low, they are still the leading cause of maternal death in the first trimester.

In an ectopic pregnancy, the gestation can grow and take its blood supply from the place it has implanted. This can eventually cause organ rupture, especially if it's located inside the fallopian tube since the tube is not designed to expand in such a way.

The Centers for Disease Control and Prevention started recording statistics for ectopic pregnancies in 1970. By 1992, they had recorded 108,800. In 1970, there were around 35 deaths per year, while by 1992, there were less than three. Still, ectopic pregnancies remain serious and strides have been taken to improve the ability to make earlier diagnoses. The earlier a diagnosis is made, the better chance there is to preserve the fallopian tubes. This is important since it helps to preserve fertility.

Though there are far fewer cases where ectopic pregnancy is life-threatening - there are more cases of ectopic pregnancy reported today than ever before. The principal reason for this is that, thanks to modern technology, it's easier to detect them. A diagnosis is made using transvaginal ultrasounds and blood work, as we'll talk about later. In the past, many ectopic pregnancies occurred and were simply reabsorbed into the woman's body and she probably never even knew she was pregnant. No treatment was needed. These days, this still happens in some cases. If you're not having any symptoms and your hCG levels are not rising your doctor might put you under what is termed "expectant management." When this happens, you'll be monitored and if anything changes, then medical intervention will be used. It's a less invasive approach then therapy or surgery.

In the past, treatment for an ectopic pregnancy was limited to surgery. Now, however, depending on where the pregnancy is located there are several options and the approach depends on symptoms, size, and hCG levels. It's possible that the doctor will take a "wait and see" approach mentioned above if there isn't any pain or bleeding present. However, if you're symptomatic, there is tissue visible on an ultrasound and blood work shows hormone levels are rising then more invasive medical procedures are probably going to be necessary. In this situation, either medication might be offered or it might be more suitable to turn to surgery. There are three different types of surgery, including laparoscopy, laparotomy, and abdominal surgery. All three have their benefits, although laparoscopy is often the preferred method since it has minimal recovery time.

Many women do successfully go on to have subsequent intrauterine pregnancies, although there is an elevated risk that they too will be ectopic. The risk factor is partly dependent on the cause of the first ectopic pregnancy. If there was extensive scar damage to the fallopian tubes that caused the first ectopic pregnancy then that risk will remain for any subsequent pregnancies. Other risk factors can increase the likelihood of ectopic pregnancies as well, such as age, smoking, and a history of sexually transmitted infections such as Chlamydia.

Luckily, even if you had a fallopian tube removed or repaired during treatment this does not seem to affect your fertility too drastically. Even with only one tube remaining, it's still possible to successfully conceive, as long as the remaining tube is healthy and functioning.

Chapter 1: What is an ectopic pregnancy?

In a normal, healthy pregnancy, the fetus develops in the inside of a woman's womb, or uterus. However, in an ectopic pregnancy, the fertilized egg attaches to a place outside of the uterus and the embryo begins developing in a place where it shouldn't be forming. The word "ectopic" actually means "out of place."

How common are ectopic pregnancies?

Ectopic pregnancies are relatively uncommon. In the United States they occur in around 2 out of every 100 pregnancies, or approximately 1-2% of all pregnancies according to data from the US Centers for Disease Control and Prevention (CDC) while in the UK they occur in about 1 in every 90 pregnancies.

In the past thirty years, however, they have become increasingly more common. Some professionals in the medical field think this is due to an increase in certain risk factors, including infertility treatments and a rise in sexually transmitted diseases and infections. Although the infections and diseases themselves do not directly increase the chance of having an ectopic pregnancy, they can leave behind adhesions and this can increase the risk.

Although in the UK the mortality from ectopic pregnancies has now fallen to about 0.2 per 100 ectopic pregnancies and in the US deaths occur to less than 1 out of 2500 cases, most of the deaths occur to women who have not sought medical treatment from the beginning of their pregnancies. Since ectopic pregnancies can be caught very early on, with standard medical care they are not as dangerous and life-threatening as they once were, although they still need to be taken very seriously.

Misdiagnosed ectopic pregnancies

Every year, women suffer from misdiagnosed ectopic pregnancies. At one time, it was suspected that as many as 40-50% of ectopic pregnancies were misdiagnosed when women first got to their doctors or emergency departments (BC Kaplan, 1996). Some women with ectopic pregnancies were sent away with diagnoses of viruses or even flu.

In addition, a pseudo-gestational sac, which is a fluid-filled sac, can show up on an ultrasound and appear to be a real gestational sac when it is not. For women with ectopic pregnancies, this can be very dangerous as it makes diagnosis harder. This makes blood work even more crucial.

Conversely, a study carried out in 1996 claimed that close to 50% of all pregnancies being treated as ectopic at that time were, in fact, viable. In 2002, an additional study by the Center for Reproductive Medicine and Surgery at the University of Pennsylvania Medical Center was published in *Obstetrics and Gynecology* and reported that as many as 40% of pregnancies diagnosed as ectopic *at that time* turned out to be viable.

In 2013, a paper entitled *Diagnostic Criteria for Nonviable Pregnancy Early in the First Trimester* in the *New England Journal of Medicine* by Dr. Peter Doubilet argued that these cases are not rare and continue on today. In this paper, researchers pointed out that the criteria that are often used to diagnose an ectopic pregnancy, including hCG levels (otherwise known as the "pregnancy hormone") might be outdated. The scientists involved in this study confirmed that their recent research, including studies conducted at the Brigham Hospital, demonstrated that the level that was defined twenty years ago as being a viable pregnancy is no longer reliable for ruling out a healthy pregnancy. It was the recommendation of this study not to treat women based on historic recommended hCG levels, since they could be prone to error (Goldberg, 2013).

Because the early symptoms of an ectopic pregnancy can be strikingly similar to those of an intrauterine pregnancy, it's often difficult to know that you have an ectopic pregnancy until it either deteriorates or you go in for your first prenatal appointment and it's discovered through blood work or ultrasound. This, along with the fact that ectopic pregnancy can mimic other medical conditions such as gastroenteritis and even appendicitis, is one of the reasons why it can be misdiagnosed and missed. If you *have* been diagnosed with an ectopic pregnancy then it's important to learn the signs and symptoms of a deteriorating ectopic pregnancy, especially if your doctor has put you on *expectant management* as a course of treatment.

Being informed and listening to your body is important as is being able to communicate with your doctor and voice your concerns about your symptoms. This will be crucial to getting the proper tests and procedures.

If you're experiencing ectopic symptoms and your doctor confirms that diagnosis, then treatment may be started, usually injections of Methotrexate. Most doctors today will monitor a woman over several days, up to a week, and take more than one blood test to see if the hCG levels are rising and do more than one ultrasound, especially if the gestation is early, *before* treatment to ensure that the pregnancy is actually ectopic. If you feel like you are receiving treatment too early you can of course seek a second opinion.

Chapter 2: What causes an ectopic pregnancy?

After receiving the diagnosis of an ectopic pregnancy, the first thing you generally want to know is why it's happened. Sometimes, the cause of an ectopic pregnancy can't be determined at all. However, it is *usually* caused by at least one of the following:

- Scar tissue or adhesions from an infection or previous surgery

- Infection or inflammation of the fallopian tube

- An abnormality in the fallopian tube

Since most ectopic pregnancies occur within the fallopian tubes, they play the biggest roles. If there are adhesions in them, or they become inflamed, then the egg and sperm can't travel through them like they're supposed to. As a result, they can become partially blocked. In some cases, they can even become completely blocked. This increases the chances of an ectopic pregnancy developing since the embryo can implant within the tube rather than inside the uterus. A prior infection or surgery can cause scar tissue to develop and this, too, can hinder the movement of the egg if it grows over the tube. Sometimes, a birth defect or abnormal growths on the fallopian tube can cause it to be misshapen, and this can also increase the risk of developing an ectopic pregnancy.

The fallopian tubes

The fallopian tubes are small and hollow and lie next to the ovaries. Inside, they have cilia, which are small hair-like projections that propel semen to the uterus. Closer to the uterus, the muscular wall gets a little thicker. Every month one of the ovaries produces an egg. This is drawn into one of the fallopian tubes and is deposited at the end, away from the uterus. Later, if intercourse happens at the right time, it might meet a sperm within the tube. This will fertilize the egg and the egg will then work its way up to tube to the uterus.

Most ectopic pregnancies occur within the fallopian tubes. Despite the fact that they do so much work, they are actually fairly delicate and fragile and it is easy for them to become damaged, especially if there is inflammation or infection involved. Sometimes, transporting a developing embryo can be thwarted and motion can be stopped in the tube. Even though the embryo isn't in the uterus, it can continue to grow and develop a placenta, right there in the tube where it stopped.

In an ideal situation, the egg implants itself in the uterus, in the endometrium, and eventually becomes a baby. However, in an ectopic pregnancy, something goes wrong along the way.

About adhesions

Adhesions are harmful because they can block the fallopian tubes. Anything that can cause an inflammatory response such as surgery, endometriosis, or an infection (including Pelvic Inflammatory Disease or a ruptured appendix) can cause the formation of adhesions.

What causes adhesions to form?

The organs in the stomach and pelvic region are wrapped in a clear membrane called the peritoneum. If there is any trauma, injury, or infection in this area, or if surgery is performed, then adhesions can form.

Adhesions can form due to:

Ovarian Surgery: Ovaries are the most common site for adhesions to form, more often than not resulting due to surgery to remove ovarian cysts.

Endometriosis Surgery: In endometriosis, pieces of the endometrial tissue implant outside the uterus. This can cause inflammation and adhesions. The tissue is often removed through surgery.

Myomectomy: A myomectomy is often used to remove fibroids from the uterus. Adhesions can form along the incision line on the uterus as a complication.

Reconstructive Tubal Surgery: The fallopian tubes can become blocked by adhesions and scar tissue. Unfortunately, removing these with surgery can bring on the formation of new adhesions.

Adhesions commonly affect women who suffer from pelvic inflammatory disease (PID) and other sexually transmitted diseases (STDs).

Adhesions can also form due to:

Trauma: The natural healing process from pelvic and abdominal surgery is a contributor to the formation of adhesions.

Ischemia: During surgery, blood flow can be disrupted due to blood clotting, the tying of stitches, or tissue cutting. Ischemia, or reduction of blood flow to the tissues, may occur and this can cause the formation of adhesions.

Foreign Objects: Very occasionally foreign objects such as talcum powder from surgical gloves, lint, and even stitches can find their way into the body during a surgery. These can cause inflammation that can lead to adhesions. It's important to stress that this is incredibly unlikely to have happened to you but if you're had a previous surgery then it is a possibility, albeit a remote one.

Inflammation: Endometriosis and PID can cause inflammation, leading to adhesion formation.

Scar tissue vs adhesions

Often, in talking about ectopic pregnancy, you'll hear the words "scar tissue" and "adhesions" and you might wonder what they mean or if they can be used interchangeably. Scar tissue and adhesions are both similar, yet they are formed for different reasons. Scar tissue occurs as the result of tissue that has been damaged and then healed. On the other hand, adhesions are a kind of scar tissue that forms within tissue that joins parts of the body. Adhesions can occur due to infection and inflammation and surgery. Conversely, scar tissue usually results from wounds such as cuts and surgical incisions.

In some literature on ectopic pregnancy, scar tissue and adhesions are used interchangeably so these terms are not something that you should get hung up on. For the purpose of this book, however, we will stick to the term "adhesions."

Where can the adhesions form?

Pelvic adhesions can form between any two tissue surfaces in the pelvic or abdominal region. They can be found in the bowel, bladder, uterus, ovaries, and fallopian tubes. Tubal surgery, including tubal ligation, can cause adhesions to form either inside or outside of the tubes. They can also form on the ends of the tubes, called the "fimbria." The fimbria, which are like tiny feathers and brush the egg into the tube, can become stuck together. In addition, tubal adhesions can also block the tube and this can cause an ectopic pregnancy since the egg and sperm can't move through it and the developing embryo will become implanted within it.

Endometriosis and adhesions

Endometriosis affects adhesions in several ways. Endometriosis is the irregular growth of cells that is similar to the cells that form the inside of the uterus. These cells can grow anywhere including outside of the uterus and on the fallopian tubes. The cells of the endometriosis attach themselves to tissue outside the uterus and are called "endometriosis implants". These implants are most frequently discovered on the ovaries, fallopian tubes, and the outer surfaces of the uterus. The existence of endometriosis can entail masses of tissue or adhesions within the pelvic region that may distort the fallopian tubes or cause them to narrow, or even block them off altogether.

Common risk factors

Even though sometimes an ectopic pregnancy simply occurs and the doctor can't determine the "why" there *are* some common risk factors that do make some women more prone to developing ectopic pregnancies than others. The following is an overview of these and why they increase the risk of an egg implanting outside of the uterus.

Endometriosis and adenomyosis

A history of endometriosis and adenomyosis can pose a threat when it comes to ectopic pregnancies. The tissue, and scar tissue that can develop from surgeries to reduce the endometriosis, can affect the fallopian tubes, as previously discussed.

Adenomyosis is similar to endometriosis in that it concerns endometrial tissue, the tissue that normally lines the uterus, except in this case it grows into the muscular wall of the uterus. Most of the time, this affects older women and doesn't happen until after menopause. However, it can affect women in their 20s and 30s and is a risk factor for ectopic pregnancies since it increases the chance of adhesions.

Ectopic pregnancy and IUDs (Mirena)

It is very rare for women to get pregnant if they have an intrauterine device (IUD) but if it does occur then the chances of having an ectopic pregnancy are higher than normal. In the past, there was a higher rate of the progesterone IUD causing ectopic pregnancies than for those women who weren't using any form of contraception at all. However, the contemporary copper IUD doesn't increase the risk of ectopic pregnancy. Still, if a woman does conceive with an IUD in place, it is more likely to be ectopic. The occurrence of ectopic pregnancies with IUD use is 3-4%.

There have been some specific concerns over Mirena. Less than 8 in 1,000 women (0.8%) become pregnant over the course of the 5 years using this form of IUD. It is still on the market, although it does list ectopic pregnancy as a complication of becoming pregnant while using it.

Although an IUD in and of itself doesn't cause the pregnancy to be ectopic, if a pregnancy does occur whilst an IUD is in place it can prevent the egg from implanting inside the uterus (since that's what its job is). On the other hand, since an IUD is used to prevent pregnancies, your chances of having an ectopic pregnancy, or any pregnancy at all, is considerably lower than it would be if you didn't have it in place. Your chances of ectopic pregnancy is not increased if you had an IUD in the past and have had it removed.

The morning after pill

There was concern that the "morning after pill" or levonorgestrel (Plan B) could be a risk factor for ectopic pregnancies. However, the studies appear to be inconclusive on this front. Some studies don't show any link between this and ectopic pregnancies (Vinson DR, 2003) while others show a 10 fold increase if the morning after pill fails to work. However, the morning after pill generally only fails to work when it is used incorrectly; ie, it is used outside of its intended timeframe.

Previous pelvic surgery

Having a surgery in the pelvic region in the past, especially where the fallopian tubes are involved, can increase the chances of having an ectopic pregnancy. Some women, for example, have surgery to reverse a tubal ligation (they had their tubes tied in the past and now they wish to have that surgery reversed) or to correct a problem that could have been caused by a birth defect. It has been discovered that 35-50% of women who conceive after having a tubal ligation are reported to experience an ectopic pregnancy. Women under the age of 35 and those who underwent electrocautery are at a higher risk (Peterson HB, 1997).

In a 1992 study conducted by the First Department of Obstetrics and Gynecology at the University of Athens in Greece, it was discovered that all kinds of previous pelvic surgeries increased the chances of an ectopic pregnancy 9 fold.

Surgery itself doesn't necessarily increase the likelihood of having an ectopic pregnancy, but it can often leave behind scar tissue and the scar tissue is the actual risk factor. Other kinds of pelvic or abdominal surgery can also increase the risk, such as an appendectomy and gallbladder removal, but not as much as surgery that affects the fallopian tubes.

A previous ectopic pregnancy

Unfortunately having had one previous ectopic pregnancy does mean there is a 10-20% likelihood of having another one.

The greater increase of having a subsequent ectopic pregnancy is based in part on why the first one occurred. If the risk factors are still present (there are still adhesions present, she still has inflammation, etc.) then the risk factors will not go down. Sometimes, of course, the reason why the first ectopic pregnancy occurred is unknown.

History of pelvic inflammatory disease (PID)

Studies show that the risk of an ectopic pregnancy in women who have a history of PID is 6 times greater than those without (J Paavonen 2008).

The most common cause of PID is a sexually transmitted infection (STI) like Chlamydia, especially if the STI went untreated. Chlamydia can cause inflammation within the fallopian tubes, and this can damage the small hairs that carry the eggs down the tubes. If the eggs get stuck in one of the tubes, an ectopic pregnancy can occur since the implantation can occur within the tube instead of within the uterus.

Since some STIs such as gonorrhea or Chlamydia often have no symptoms, you might not know that you have one unless you are tested by your doctor. If you did have Chlamydia and it was treated, the bacteria could still have led to scarring within the tubes. However, it's possible for one tube to be affected and not the other. If you've had an ectopic pregnancy, and have a history of an STI, unfortunately the only way to determine if the STI caused the ectopic pregnancy would be to have the tube removed and see if there are any signs of scarring that could be associated with Chlamydia or another STI. Most women would of course not choose to have a fallopian tube removed so this is something that can only be determined when a tube has been removed during surgery because it is too badly damaged to be repaired.

Having had multiple sexual partners is considered a risk factor, too, but only in the sense that in can increase the chances of developing an STI or PID.

There are additional organisms that cause PID, such as salpingitis (an infection and inflammation in the fallopian tubes). This can increase the risk of ectopic pregnancy 4-fold.

The risk of tubal damage can increase after each successive episode of PID. For example, it increases 13% after 1 episode, 35% after 2 episodes, and 75% after 3 episodes.

The DES drug

If your mother took the drug DES (*diethylstilbestrol*) while she was pregnant with you then you might suffer from damaged fallopian tubes or abnormalities of your uterus. These issues also pose a risk factor. DES was a medication offered to women in the past to keep them from miscarrying while pregnant. However, DES was removed in 1971 from the US market so it's unlikely that this applies to most women (Hoover RN, 2011). However, it remained available in other countries so there is a slight chance that your mother may have taken it. This is something that you might want to ask when looking at your own medical history.

Age

Women who are 35 years of age or older when they conceive are at a higher risk, with the highest rate occurring to those women who are between the ages of 35 and 44. The reasons for this are unknown, but might have to do with more opportunity for damage to occur to the fallopian tubes or a greater likelihood of having been exposed to a pelvic infection.

Smoking

Smoking may elevate the chances of an ectopic pregnancy forming. Some studies have shown that women smokers are 1.6 to 3.5 times more likely to have an ectopic pregnancy than nonsmokers. It's possible that smoking might damage the fallopian tubes and make them unable to function properly, thus causing the risk to increase. Smoking might also delay ovulation and alter uterine motility. However, there hasn't been a specific study published yet that has determined a reason why smoking might affect the incidence of ectopic pregnancies.

Other birth control methods

Some studies have shown that if you become pregnant while taking certain oral contraceptives, like those that are progestin-only (mini pill), there is an increased risk of ectopic pregnancy. However, studies are vague as to how much the risk is increased or if there is an increased risk at all.

Some literature suggests that the risk of an ectopic pregnancy is decreased using the mini pill since the overall risk of ovulation is. On the other hand, if pregnancy does occur while on the mini pill, then there is a 5% higher risk that the pregnancy might be an ectopic one, possibly because the progestin (synthetic progesterone) can modify the tubal function and slow down the rate of ovum transport.

Certain fertility procedures

As we've established, problems with fertility are often caused by damaged fallopian tubes. The damaged fallopian tubes themselves can be a risk factor, but some fertility treatments can also put a woman at a higher risk for an ectopic pregnancy.

Inducing ovulation with clomiphene citrate (commonly known as Clomid) or injectable gonadotropin therapy has been connected with a 4-fold increase in the risk of ectopic pregnancy (SN Tripathy, 2013). It is possible that multiple eggs and high hormone levels may increase the risk in this scenario.

Some fertility procedures can also increase the chances. For instance, if a fertilized egg has been inserted into a fallopian tube then there is the slight chance that it might implant there rather than in the uterus. In most cases, however, this will only happen if there is damage to the tube that keeps the egg from traveling.

It has also been found that the risk of ectopic pregnancy or a heterotopic pregnancy (having both an intrauterine and ectopic pregnancy at the same time) does increase when women use assisted reproductive techniques like in vitro fertilization (IVF) or gamete intrafallopian transfer (GIFT) (Dor J, 1991). In GIFT, the sperm and egg are combined outside of the body and then inserted into the fallopian tubes where they are fertilized within the body. Sometimes, rather than moving up the tube, the egg implants within the fallopian tubes and an ectopic pregnancy develops.

Concerning in vitro, in one study, the rate of ectopic pregnancies was 4.5%. Other studies have shown that up to 1% of IVF or GIFT pregnancies can result in a heterotopic gestation (Svare JA, 1994). In a study carried out by the Catholic Medical Center of Brooklyn and Queens in New York, women who had luteal phase defects (disruptions in their monthly menstrual cycles) were shown to have a higher ectopic pregnancy rates than women whose infertility were caused by anovulation (when ovulation effectively doesn't take place).

Are ectopic pregnancies hereditary?

Ectopic pregnancies are not hereditary. Most studies show that they occur due to some type of damage to the reproductive organs, some of which could be attributed to congenital birth defects.

Although there is a possibility that women whose mothers took DES, a synthetic non-steroidal estrogen pill that was meant to stop miscarriages from happening, this is not a hereditary issue but a chemical one. Most women aren't at any higher risk of having an ectopic pregnancy even if their mothers had one as well.

Can an ectopic pregnancy be prevented?

Most ectopic pregnancies cannot be prevented at this time since, for the most part, it is unknown why the majority of them formed in the first place. However, you can take certain measures to lower your risk factors. Some steps that you might want to take if you plan on having a subsequent pregnancy to lower your risk factors include:

- Stop smoking

- If you suffer from endometriosis, have any scar tissue removed

- Get tested and treated for any possible STIs

- Always wear protection when engaging in sexual intercourse with a new partner

- If you take the morning after pill, take it within the designated timeframe (up to five days or 120 hours after unprotected sex)

- Identify the risks and symptoms of pelvic inflammatory disease and seek treatment from your healthcare provider to avoid scarring and inflammation

- Have regular checkups with your gynecologist, including testing for sexually transmitted diseases and pap smears.

Chapter 3: Types of ectopic pregnancies

Ectopic pregnancies can show up in different parts of the pelvic and abdominal regions, although tubal pregnancies are the most common, accounting for 80-95% for all ectopic pregnancies.

Four different segments of the fallopian tubes can be affected in an ectopic pregnancy: ampulla, isthmus, fimbrial, and interstitial. If a pregnancy is located in any of these parts of the fallopian tubes, it's still considered a tubal pregnancy. Ampullary pregnancies are the most common, occurring in more than 80% of all ectopic pregnancies. The ampulla is the second segment of the fallopian tube and curls over the ovary. The isthmic segment is a narrow muscular segment which is closest to the uterus and sees 12% of the ectopic pregnancies. The fimbria is the fringe of tissue at the opening of the tubes near the ovaries. Around 5% of ectopic pregnancies occur here. Lastly, the interstitial segment passes through the uterine muscle into the uterine cavity and 2% of ectopic pregnancies can be implanted here, making it the rarest of the tubal locations.

Other sites an ectopic pregnancy can be located are:

In the abdomen: 1%

In or on the ovary: 0.2%

On the cervix: 0.2%

Tubal pregnancy

Most of the time, an ectopic pregnancy involves the fallopian tubes. Sometimes however, the embryo can get dislodged and will move, causing an abdominal ectopic pregnancy.

The fallopian tubes are designed to carry eggs and sperm, not a developing embryo. When an embryo starts developing in the fallopian tube, it can be a very serious matter. Not only does the pregnancy become unviable, it can also cause complications for the woman's health.

Fallopian tubes are not able to stretch wide enough to accommodate a developing fetus and, after a certain amount of time, they may rupture. This can cause intense pain and internal bleeding and is a serious medical emergency.

Atypical ectopic pregnancies

Ectopic pregnancies that do not occur within the fallopian tubes are considered to be "atypical" ectopic pregnancies. The atypical locations include the ovarian, cervical, interstitial (also called cornual), abdominal, and those that can form within Caesarean scar tissue.

Interstitial pregnancy

An interstitial pregnancy, or cornual pregnancy, is also essentially a tubal pregnancy and occurs when the fertilized egg implants in the part of the fallopian tube that's buried deep within the uterine wall. Although this is a tubal pregnancy, they only account for 2% of the ectopic pregnancies and are therefore rare so they're considered atypical. They can also be tricky to diagnose since on ultrasounds they appear to be inside the uterus. These kinds of ectopic pregnancies are especially dangerous since they can develop for longer without detection and then rupture, causing severe complications.

On an ultrasound, interstitial pregnancies may show an unconventional gestational sac that may even appear to be inside the uterus.

Treatment depends on size and stability. Medication is sometimes the first course of action, although surgery is more common and involves a procedure to remove the pregnancy from the uterine wall. However, this is risky for those who wish to conceive in the future since it could result in the uterus being weaker than before. However, many women do go on to have successful pregnancies after having this kind of surgery.

Abdominal

In most cases, ectopic pregnancies in the abdominal region are thought to have started in the fallopian tubes and then separated and moved up into the abdomen. They account for around 1% to 1.4% of all ectopic pregnancies. Abdominal pregnancies can remain undetected for many weeks and even exhibit symptoms of normal, healthy pregnancies into the first trimester, depending on which organ they have attached to.

There are occasionally news stories about abdominal ectopic pregnancies that are later delivered successfully. However, though possible, this is extremely rare and very dangerous, as we will later discuss.

In or on the ovary

An ectopic pregnancy located on or in the ovary accounts for about 0.2% of all ectopic pregnancies. For an egg implanted here, surgery is usually required, involving at least a partial removal of the affected ovary. Even with a partial removal, the ovary can nevertheless continue to produce eggs so fertility is preserved.

In the cervix

Cervical pregnancies account for around 0.2% of all ectopic pregnancies. One of the leading risk factors for an egg implanting on the cervix is prior surgical trauma, including a Dilation and Curettage (D & C). Because the cervix is vascular in nature, it's considered very serious if an egg implants on it. In the past, if a rupture occurred, an emergency hysterectomy would have been the only option. Now with more visibility using transvaginal ultrasounds, ectopic pregnancy can usually be caught early on and cervical ectopic pregnancies can, in most cases, be managed using Methotrexate or potassium chloride.

Heterotopic Pregnancy

A heterotopic pregnancy occurs when there are two embryos: a viable pregnancy within the uterus and an ectopic pregnancy outside of the uterus at the same time. This only happens in less than 1-2% of ectopic pregnancies, making it extremely rare. The survival rate of the uterine fetus of an ectopic pregnancy is around 70%, however, which is positive.

Where twins are concerned, in a heterotopic pregnancy, it is possible for the co-existing intrauterine twin to survive. This occurs in about 30% of diagnosed cases of heterotopic pregnancies, despite the woman being treated surgically.

In the scar of a caesarean section

It is extremely uncommon for an ectopic pregnancy to be located within a C-section scar, although it can happen. It is thought to occur in around 1 in 18,000 cases although the frequency might be increasing due to the number of elective C-sections that are occurring today.

When an ectopic pregnancy occurs in a C-section scar, the egg implants within the scar tissue itself. A thin suction catheter is generally passed through the cervix to remove the pregnancy if the pregnancy is very early. Usually, no other treatment is required, although sometimes a stitch might be needed within the cervix to stop any bleeding that might be present.

Successful ectopic pregnancies

Nearly all ectopic pregnancies are considered nonviable. Although not all ectopic pregnancies require surgery for treatment, all are considered at risk of eventual rupture and resulting hemorrhage, so they are closely managed. Tubal pregnancies are not considered viable in any manner.

In extremely rare cases, around 1 in one million, a pregnancy can be implanted in the abdomen and be delivered successfully. However, this poses an extreme risk to the woman's health, as well as to the baby's. In an abdominal pregnancy, the placenta rests on one of the abdominal organs or on the peritoneum. It also require adequate blood supply from another source, usually from the bowels, kidneys, livers, or aorta. The baby is usually delivered very early in order to help ensure mother and baby's health, but even then maternal morbidity and mortality is high since it can be difficult to detach the placenta from the organs and this can cause hemorrhaging.

There have been no official studies carried out on incidents involving successful abdominal pregnancies so the rates are unknown.

Chapter 4: Symptoms of an ectopic pregnancy

Symptoms of an ectopic pregnancy can appear very early in a pregnancy and may vary depending on the woman and where the pregnancy is located. However, some women don't have any symptoms at all and sometimes they mimic ordinary pregnancy symptoms. The important thing is that if you've been diagnosed with an ectopic pregnancy already, it's possible for the pregnancy to deteriorate very rapidly so you must know what signs to look out for.

The symptoms of ectopic pregnancy are especially important because they'll help determine the course of treatment. If you're not experiencing a lot of symptoms, or the ones you're experiencing are manageable, then it's possible that your doctor will put you under something that's called "expectant management." In this treatment course, you'll be closely watched and monitored in the hope that your body will naturally reabsorb the pregnancy without any surgical or medicinal intervention.

Early symptoms of ectopic pregnancies

In the beginning of an ectopic pregnancy, different women experience different things. There are actually several possible scenarios and we'll go over each one.

Some women discover that they're pregnant by taking a home pregnancy test. For the first few weeks of their pregnancy, they have what would be characterized as "typical" pregnancy symptoms that include nausea, vomiting, and tender breasts. When they go in for their first prenatal appointment, however, and get their blood work, their doctor might discover that their hCG hormone levels aren't as high as expected, based on gestation age and date of last menstrual cycle. The doctor might then send the woman home and ask her to come back in another day or two to have the blood work repeated. If, by then, the levels haven't doubled as anticipated then he or she might do a transvaginal ultrasound to look for an egg sac (keeping in mind that in the early weeks of a pregnancy it might still be difficult to see anything).

At this point, she may or may not be feeling anything "off." To her, the pregnancy might have felt as though it was progressing as normal so the news that the embryo was implanted within her fallopian tubes and not within her uterus would be a complete surprise.

On the other hand, some women deteriorate very rapidly, almost before they even realized they were pregnant. They might experience vaginal bleeding that starts out as brown and gradually turns red, stabbing or cramping pain in their right side, light headedness, confusion, and even lose consciousness.

An ectopic pregnancy can start out progressing as a normal pregnancy, with little to no symptoms, making it difficult to distinguish it from anything other than being a intrauterine 'normal' pregnancy. Although some women do experience nausea, vomiting, and spotting, these are also common in intrauterine pregnancies and therefore indistinguishable from an ectopic one.

Some women can experience abdominal pain as the embryo grows, especially if it is located within a fallopian tube, but many pregnant women also experience something called round ligament pain during the first trimester so even this symptom is not always telling of an ectopic pregnancy. The pain associated with an ectopic pregnancy, however, is usually located on one side – though this doesn't always happen, because not all ectopic pregnancies are tubal in nature.

It is not until an ectopic pregnancy really starts to deteriorate that the symptoms begin to distinguish themselves from a normal pregnancy and these are the symptoms that you should become familiar with, especially if your doctor has taken an expectant management approach with you.

A deteriorating ectopic pregnancy

After you have been diagnosed with an ectopic pregnancy, your doctor will determine the best course of action for you. This will be based on where your pregnancy is located and what your symptoms are. Most doctors like to take the least invasive approach, but if there are signs of internal bleeding or if you're in a lot of pain then surgery will more than likely be the best course of action. If the pregnancy does not appear to be growing rapidly, then it's possible that the doctor will take the expectant management route in hopes that the pregnancy will be absorbed by the body or use medication known as Methotrexate.

If you do experience any symptoms that concern you, especially abdominal pain or vaginal bleeding, it's imperative to take them seriously because they could be signs that the ectopic pregnancy is deteriorating. A deteriorating pregnancy could mean the rupture of a fallopian tube or of any organ that the pregnancy is attached to, such as the ovary.

The rupture of a fallopian tube is considered an obstetric emergency and it's important to notify your doctor as soon as possible in order to get an accurate diagnosis so that you can get treated just in case there is a problem.

The signs of a deteriorating ectopic pregnancy can come when you're being treated either with expectant management or Methotrexate or before you've actually been diagnosed with an ectopic pregnancy.

Two things that you want to be on the lookout for when it comes to a deteriorating ectopic pregnancy include: signs of rupture and signs of shock. Both come with their own set of symptoms.

Signs of rupture

- Abdominal or pelvic pain: Signs of rupture include sharp, stabbing pain in the stomach or pelvic region. Most women describe this as pain on one side of the stomach. However, the pain doesn't have to be limited to one side. It can start on one side, and then spread to the other in a radiating type of pain. The pain can be intense, and cause nausea and vomiting. It is not alleviated by lying down, taking medicine, or participating in any relaxing activities such as taking a warm bath or using a heating pad.

- Vaginal bleeding: Vaginal spotting or bleeding is a common symptom of ectopic pregnancies. In a rupture, however, the bleeding may be very heavy. It has been described as the color of prune juice. If the bleeding is heavy enough to soak through a sanitary napkin in an hour then it's important to contact your local emergency department or have someone take you there on your behalf.

- Shoulder tip pain: Shoulder tip pain is one of the most important symptoms of an ectopic pregnancy and something that you should take very seriously. Shoulder tip pain is generally caused by internal bleeding which can irritate the diaphragm when you breathe in and out. Pain in the shoulder, especially upon lying down, can mean that the pregnancy has ruptured. In this case, it's imperative that medical care is sought immediately. The pain itself probably means that internal bleeding is occurring and causing the nerves that lead to your shoulder area to be irritated.

Signs of shock

Signs of shock can include: clammy skin, dizziness, fainting, and a racing pulse. Some women report that before they went into shock they felt light-headed, confused and disoriented. Although not all women lose consciousness, others do.

Many women later talk about "collapsing" and getting what they described as "tunnel vision" that came out of nowhere while they were sitting, standing, or walking. Low blood pressure, sometimes caused by internal and external blood loss can cause some of these symptoms.

If you're experiencing signs of shock then call 911 in the US or 999 for the ambulance service in the UK.

It's important to listen to your body. If you feel like something is wrong, then try waiting for about an hour and assess yourself to see if things are improving or getting worse. If you're in pain, taking a Tylenol or Paracetamol and lying down in a quiet place and relaxing is a good start. If, after half an hour to an hour, you're not feeling any better, then it might be a good idea to call your doctor.

Chapter 5: Treatment options

In the past, surgery was the only treatment option for ectopic pregnancies and abdominal surgery was the only type of surgery that was offered. The recovery time was long and the hospital stay could be as long as a week. These days, things have changed. Although an ectopic pregnancy is a serious medical condition, a laparoscopic surgery to have a fallopian tube repaired can be considered an out-patient surgery in some hospitals (although in many it's still at least a one night stay).

There are three main therapeutic options for treatment in ectopic pregnancy and they are as follows:

- Expectant management

- Methotrexate

- Surgery

The selection of these treatment options is based in part on how far along the pregnancy is and where it is located. Some ectopic pregnancies will resolve on their own and no intervention is needed. However, other pregnancies have life-threatening bleeding present and will require urgent surgery due to the risk of rupture. Every case is a little different.

Expectant Management

As we've mentioned there is always the possibility that the body will naturally absorb an ectopic pregnancy. This is actually an ideal option since it requires no medical intervention such as surgery or medication and is therefore easier on your body. If a doctor believes that this may be possible with your ectopic pregnancy then you could be placed on 'expectant management' and watched to see what happens with your pregnancy next.

Women who are candidates for successful expectant management don't have any symptoms, or have symptoms that aren't interfering with their daily lives, and have shown no evidence of rupture or hemodynamic instability (when the cardiovascular system can't sustain itself without mechanical support or the use of medications). If there is bleeding present, it should only be seen as light spotting, indicating old blood. (Bright red blood would indicate that it is fresh.) There shouldn't be any shoulder pain or sharp pain in the side, which could indicate rupture.

If your doctor thinks expectant management is right for you they will ensure that you:

- Understand there is a risk of rupture and hemorrhage

- Have decreasing levels hCG, which suggests the body is reabsorbing the ectopic pregnancy

- Be able to see the doctor for regular checkups

If your doctor chooses this option for you then your pregnancy would be managed by following you very, very closely. Doctor visits would be critical on a regular basis since tubal ruptures could still occur, even with low and declining serum levels of β-hCG. Declining levels would indicate that the body is absorbing the pregnancy, but as long as the embryo is still implanted within the fallopian tubes (or on another organ) there is still a health risk present until all of the tissue is gone.

In most ectopic pregnancies, there is never a heartbeat since the babies do not get the chance to grow. Since the egg implanted outside of the uterus, it didn't find a good blood supply source and the trophoblasts (specialized cells of the placenta) more or less 'burrow' into the walls of whatever structure the egg stuck to. For some women, as the hCG levels stop rising, the trophoblast cells and tissue naturally stop dividing. What occurs at this point depends on the individual woman.

In some cases, the tissue will shrink and then this is when it will be reabsorbed back into the body. This is a natural process, but it doesn't happen immediately, however, and can actually take weeks and even months to completely finish. Sometimes, during the process, the fallopian tube can still become blocked by the tissue as the body is trying to absorb it. If this occurs, medication may be needed or surgery may be required, depending on the severity of the blockage and the symptoms.

There is a risk that goes along with expectant management. The biggest risk, of course, is that the body won't absorb the pregnancy or dispel it naturally and that rupture will occur. Approximately 25% of women who are expectantly managed end up requiring medical or surgical treatment. However, doctors *can* tell if the specialized cells of a pregnancy that produce the hCG hormone are dividing since the hCG level will go up and not down.

A good doctor will closely monitor his or her patient and advise wisely, suggesting medication or surgery when needed. Sometimes, though, an ectopic pregnancy can rupture despite low hCG levels. If you are under expectant management then it's important to alert your doctor if anything in your body changes. Let him or her know immediately if you experience any of the symptoms we've talked about. To summarize these include:

- Shoulder tip pain

- Abdominal pain (especially on one side)

- Bleeding

- Dizziness

- Lightheadedness

- Nausea

- Vomiting

- Confusion

- Disorientation

Methotrexate

A lot of unruptured ectopic pregnancies today are treated with medications, most commonly Methotrexate (Rheumatrex, Trexall). No statistics exist on how many pregnancies are treated with this medication, but more and more medical centers are offering it as an alternative to surgery.

This medication is an anti-cancer drug and kills the growing cells of the placenta, more or less inducing miscarriage of the ectopic pregnancy. Methotrexate does not start working right away; it takes several days for the cells to begin dividing. In fact, hCG levels might even go up after the first day. However, if there isn't a drop in hCG levels by at least 15% (this varies according to doctor) by the end of the week then a second dose is generally given or surgery is considered.

Methotrexate is gaining in popularity due to its high success rate and the fact that it doesn't have many adverse reactions. In most cases, only a single dose needs to be administered, although sometimes a double dose is needed since a few patients may not respond. The typical success rates for a single-dosage Methotrexate course of therapy is 88-94%. In one study, 94% of the women were successfully treated with only one dose without any adverse reactions (TG Stovall, 1992). In addition, out of the women who went on to conceive a subsequent pregnancy, 87.2% of those pregnancies were intrauterine while only 12.8% were ectopic. Similar studies had comparable results.

A double dose course of therapy has shown a somewhat stronger success rate of 91-95%. In a meta-analysis that was comprised of data from 26 trials the data showed a success rate of 92.7% (Kt Barnhart, 2003) with the multiple-dose regimen. Still, whether doctors choose to use one dose or two, the success rates are considered to be very high and many women do go on to have successful pregnancies that are intrauterine and not ectopic should they chose to conceive again.

A good candidate for Methotrexate treatment should have:

- No serious abdominal pain

- Good overall health

- Low hCG levels

- The ability to make follow-up appointments

- Hemodynamic stability

- Normal liver and renal function

There are some specific situations in which Methotrexate therapy should not be used for a patient. These include the following:

- In the existence of an intrauterine pregnancy

- If a patient has any of the following:

    o Immunodeficiency

- o Moderate or severe leukopenia, thrombocytopenia, or anemia

- o Peptic ulcer disease

- o Hepatic or renal dysfunction

- If the patient is breastfeeding

- If there is evidence of a tubal rupture.

When can I have Methotrexate?

It is most effective to take Methotrexate in the early stages of pregnancy, typically when the hCG level is below 3000<mIU/mL since the risk of rupture is higher when levels exceed this. On the other hand, where cornual ectopic pregnancies are concerned, it's not unheard of to try to treat with higher levels - if the doctor is prepared to use Methotrexate at all (cornual pregnancies are usually treated with surgery). When considering an ectopic pregnancy, doctors don't really consider the gestation as much as the size of the embryo. The rate of growth is the most important aspect of the pregnancy for determining treatment.

Are there any risks to this treatment?

Regardless to the treatment option, all women who have had an ectopic pregnancy are advised not to become pregnant for at least two menstrual cycles, preferably three. If you have had Methotrexate, this is especially important since it may have reduced the level of folate in your body.

Folate is important to ensure a baby develops in a healthy manner. A folate deficiency, for instance, could result in a greater chance of the baby having a neural tube defect such as spina bifida. Even though Methotrexate is metabolized quickly it can still affect the quality of the cells, including those of your eggs, for up to 3 or 4 months after it has been administered.

Methotrexate can also affect the way the liver works so the body must have proper time to recover before a new pregnancy begins. Before conception, it is now advised to start taking folic acid several months before trying to conceive. However, it's important to *not* start taking folic acid until the hCG levels are below 5<mIU/mL. Once the hCG levels have dropped, if you want to start trying to conceive again, start taking folic acid supplements or a multi-vitamin supplement that contains folic acid. If you've had Methotrexate treatment then it's a good idea to do a detox to help clear the toxins from your system – we give some ideas and tips for detoxing later on.

How it works

The Methotrexate dose is calculated according to your height and weight. Before it's administered, blood tests are done to check liver and kidney functions and to ensure that you're not anemic. Methotrexate is injected into a muscle. It reaches the embryo through the bloodstream. The small embryo is then reabsorbed into the body over time.

Most women do usually experience some side effects as the drug begins working. These can include:

- Cramping

- Abdominal pain

- Nausea

- Diarrhea

- Vomiting

The doctor might prescribe some anti-nausea tablets to help alleviate some of these symptoms. Some women experience bleeding which usually lasts a couple of weeks and will change from a brighter red to a darker brown and then to pink before it tapers off. There is generally no need to worry unless it's accompanied by very heavy one-sided pain and unbearable cramping that can't be alleviated with over-the-counter pain medication.

Methotrexate works by depleting the body of the essential vitamin it needs to replicate cells. Our bodies are always replicating cells. Although Methotrexate is technically short-acting, our bodies must still work hard to try to recover from the reduction of folacin. On or around the 4th day after treatment, most women feel very exhausted since the drug interferes with the essential amino acids that give us energy. It is usually easier on the body if you take things slowly for the first few weeks after taking Methotrexate, at least until you get your energy back.

For a certain amount of time, it will be important to avoid taking any non-steroidal anti-inflammatory drugs (NSAIDs) ibuprofen, aspirin, or naproxen. It's also important to avoid any multivitamins or supplements that contain folic acid as these can help the cells replicate. For at least a week or two sex should be avoided until your levels are down to less than 100<mlU/mL.

Alcohol should also be avoided since Methotrexate is metabolized in the liver the same way as alcohol. It can alter liver enzymes in the short term and traces of the drug can be found in the liver as long as 100 days after the last dose. This could make you feel sick and even potentially cause long-term damage to the liver.

At a follow-up appointment, the doctor will take blood work to check the hCG levels to ensure that the ectopic pregnancy has been reabsorbed. The test will be re-administered until the hCG levels have returned to 0.

Until the levels have reached 0, it will be important to contact the A&E or ER right away if there are any signs of rupture or shock. Signs of rupture include: shoulder pain, heavy bleeding, and severe stomach pain. Again, signs of shock include: pale, clammy skin; dizziness, fainting, weakness, and a racing pulse.

Side effects of Methotrexate

The most common side effects of Methotrexate are:

- Abdominal pain. It usually occurs during the first 2-3 days of treatment. However, since this is also a sign of a ruptured ectopic pregnancy, please report any abdominal pain to your healthcare provider.

- Vaginal bleeding or spotting

- Nausea and vomiting

- Fatigue, lightheadedness, or dizziness

Other (rare) side effects from Methotrexate include:

- Sensitivity to sunlight

- Sore throat

- Hair loss

- Inflammation of the lungs

The same as a miscarriage?

Sometimes, the bleeding that can accompany an ectopic pregnancy that is treated either with Methotrexate or with expectant management can result in heavy bleeding. Tissue or clots can be passed at this time. Some women think they are passing an embryo or placenta and this can lead them to believe that they are experiencing a miscarriage.

Although Methotrexate causes you to have a type of miscarriage, in that your body is rejecting the mass of cells that is being implanted within your body, it's important to remember you're not actually miscarrying a viable fetus. Keeping this in mind may help later on in the grieving process.

The bleeding, though heavy (and definitely a cause for worry if it's accompanied by pain on one side and signs of shock) is not actually a miscarriage. It is the passing of what is known as a "decidual cast." This decidual cast can cause confusion, and women can mistake it for the tissue of their baby.

When a woman is pregnant, the lining of the uterus is called the decidua: all of that except which is taken up by the placenta. When part of the decidua is shed it is called a decidual cast. This happens due to lack of stability of the the lining as a result of the hormones not functioning the way they should be in an ectopic pregnancy. When the hormones drop abruptly, the substances inside the uterus can shed and this material can be passed through the vagina. The tissue that is passed can appear to be white, red, gray, or pink.

Passing a decidual cast can be a very traumatic experience for a woman. It doesn't just happen in an ectopic pregnancy and can occur for a variety of other reasons, but it can be particularly difficult where an ectopic pregnancy is concerned because it can resemble a miscarriage and can intensify the feelings of loss.

The amount of this that you pass can vary, depending on how far along you were. Some women do pass a lot of tissue. Many women, who prefer doing a lot of research on their own, are shocked to find images online of decidual casts. Rest assured that these images are not what you will pass. Although there are frightening images out there, the casts break up as they pass through your system, and they actually come out in much smaller pieces. Generally, those seen in medical books, are those which have been removed through surgical procedures.

Surgical treatment

Although medication is the preferred course of treatment when expectant management is not possible, it is not always the *best* treatment. Surgery has long been the established course of treatment for ectopic pregnancies and is still the most widely used, even though it comes with its own risks.

When choosing surgery, the doctor generally does so because he or she has looked at the pregnancy and the high beta hCG levels and decided that less invasive treatments are not the right option since they might put the patient at risk. If there are symptoms present, hCG levels are still rising, or medication has failed then surgery might simply be the next option to consider.

What happens during surgery?

There are different kinds of surgery techniques to treat ectopic pregnancy. These consist of laparotomies, laparoscopies, and abdominal surgeries.

Laparotomy

In a laparotomy, an incision is made in the lower abdomen. A laparotomy is generally only used for patients who are hemodynamically unstable (the blood pressure is so low that the tissues aren't being supplied with enough oxygen and blood), have a lot of bleeding, or for those who have cornual ectopic pregnancies.

Laparoscopy

In some cases, laparoscopy is used as an investigative approach to determine the presence of an ectopic pregnancy and also used to repair organs if needed. It is also a surgical technique and can be used to remove an ectopic pregnancy. It is the most favored approach since it is less invasive. A little bit of gas is inserted into the stomach to inflate it and then a small camera is inserted inside so that the surgeon can look around.

If there is an ectopic pregnancy in the fallopian tube then a small incision can be made in the tube and the pregnancy can be removed at that time. The tube can then be left intact. Laparoscopies are not always ideal, though. If there is a lot of pelvic scar tissue and excessive blood in the abdomen or pelvis, it might not be possible to perform a laparoscopy. Sometimes, depending on how much damage has been done to the fallopian tube, the entire tube might need to be removed, or at least part of it, and this can require a different type of surgery.

A laparoscopic surgery requires general anesthesia. The surgeon will be experienced in the technique. It takes around a week to recuperate from the surgery. Although some women are up walking around later that day, it can take as long as one week for the excess gas that was inserted into your abdomen to be eliminated from your body. Many women find their arms and chest particularly uncomfortable since that seems to be where the gas rests. Constipation is also commonly felt after surgery as well, as is pain from the incision spot.

Similarly with the medication treatment, it's important to get blood tests after the surgery to monitor the hCG levels to ensure removal of the ectopic pregnancy was complete. This will continue until the levels reach 0, which usually takes a few weeks.

Abdominal Surgery

Sometimes, especially if there is extensive scar tissue in the abdomen or heavy bleeding present, laparoscopic technology may not be an option at all. This is fairly rare, but it still happens. If this occurs, then abdominal surgery may be the only surgery that is possible.

Unlike laparoscopic surgery or even a laparotomy, abdominal surgery is not an out-patient procedure and has a much longer recovery time which can be as long as 6 weeks.

General anesthesia will be administered and an ob-gyn will open the abdomen and remove the embryo, wherever it may be located. The tube may be preserved or may need to be removed, depending on the situation, which is the same as with laparoscopic surgery. Generally speaking, it takes about 6-8 weeks to completely heal afterwards. The hospital stay is anywhere from 1-4 days. Some common side effects of the surgery include abdominal pain, bloating, incision pain and tenderness, constipation, and nausea.

Salpingectomy

In some cases, if the ectopic pregnancy is located within the fallopian tube and the tube is badly damaged and can't be repaired, part of it may need to be removed. This is referred to as a partial salpingectomy, if only part of the tube is removed or a complete salpingectomy if the entire tube must be removed. It can be removed using any of the previous methods.

Salpingotomy

If there hasn't been a lot of damage to the tube then a small hole can be made in it and the embryo can be removed through the opening. The tube can then remain intact. This procedure is called a salpingotomy and is ideal since it leaves both tubes behind. If only a small portion of the tube is removed in the middle, for instance, then it can be rejoined later using microsurgery. However, it does have a drawback since it is possible that part of the pregnancy could be left behind, no matter how minimal. This happens in around 5-15% of cases and may be treated by surgically removing the tube or by using Methotrexate therapy.

As with other treatment options, patients will continue to have regular blood work to monitor their hCG levels to ensure that they're decreasing. If they're not declining as they should then Methotrexate may need to be administered.

Other surgeries

In rare cases, when an ectopic pregnancy attaches to the ovary, an oophorectomy must be performed. This is the removal of the ovary. An oophorectomy can usually be performed through a laparoscopy.

Ovarian ectopic pregnancies are rare, with risk factors being previous pelvic inflammatory disease, IUD use, endometriosis, and assisted reproductive technologies.

Interstitial pregnancy has traditionally been treated through hysterectomies since the ectopic pregnancy can be firmly implanted deep within the uterine walls and cannot always be treated effectively with Methotrexate, possibly because the embryos have increased blood supply and higher hCG levels. Occasionally, corneal resection has been used if there hasn't been a severely damaged uterus present.

If there was a badly damaged uterus then either abdominal surgery or a laparotomy would be required, although laparoscopies are becoming more and more common today in these instances.

Chapter 6: Recovering from the emotional strain

Many women find it difficult to deal with their sense of loss after discovering that they have an ectopic pregnancy. Even though ectopic pregnancies are considered early pregnancy losses, the feelings that accompany them are similar to those that women who experience miscarriages often feel. Some women feel particularly devastated because they had been trying to conceive for a long time and then to hear that the pregnancy is not only unviable but that their health might be in danger is disheartening to say the least.

In addition, in some cases surgery is involved as a course of treatment and along with surgery there is a recovery period that can be challenging and emotional in its own way. Not everyone has a strong support system and the hormone changes alone can be challenging. Many women end up feeling sad, angry, and depressed.

On top of your own feelings, your partner may also be experiencing his loss in a way that is difficult to understand. Although the two of you share the experience together and want to support one another, sometimes partners are not always able to support each other the way they want to. Your partner might feel helpless. For some couples, this kind of experience actually brings them closer together. For others, it creates a strain.

Sometimes, you might end up having flashbacks of receiving the news of your diagnosis and certain aspects of your treatment process. Some women actually develop Post Traumatic Stress Disorder and experience anxiety and even panic attacks as triggers remind them of the painful experience. They experience physical and emotional reactions to these triggers. Reliving the experience could interfere with daily activities and cause depression or anxiety.

Many women also experience numbness at times, or a feeling of an emotional void. You might feel as though you can't connect with the world around you and that you're detached from what is going on. You might feel frustrated with the people in your life and feel that they don't seem to be able to understand what you're going through and how you feel.

As with any form of grief, you could feel happy, sad, confused, angry, guilty, and even scared. You may even feel all of these at the same time as grief is now understood to be non-linear (meaning you don't move progressively from one 'stage' of grief to the next). Feeling afraid is very common, as is feeling angry. You might feel angry that your body "betrayed" you, angry at your doctor for not being able to "save" your baby (even though it wasn't medically possible), angry because you're not in charge your own body, and even angry at your partner for not being able to make things "better." Anger is an easy emotion for the human body to resort to because it's one we're comfortable with. Depression and guilt can be scary but anger can give us energy and pump up our energy, which is one of the reasons why the mind often seems to prefer it to almost anything else.

If you have other children, you might find that you suddenly feel more protective towards them. You may feel like you need to spend more time with them, or you might start worrying about them more and show concern in areas that you didn't worry about before. This might actually affect you physically as you start having trouble sleeping, worrying about whether or not they'll be safe at school or on the road or if they're breathing in their sleep.

The important thing to remember is that the reactions that you have are understandable. The experience you've been through *is* an overwhelming and traumatic one and it will take time to overcome. However, it's also important to take things one step at a time and to heal slowly. It's also important to find support where you can.

Some things you may learn along the way…

- Don't worry about feeling like you're not overcoming your grief as quickly as you would like. All you can do is take this one step at a time and there is no set time when you will feel emotionally stronger.

- Whenever a body goes from being pregnant to not being pregnant, there is a considerable shift in hormones. This *will* affect brain chemistry. Give yourself time to heal.

- Grief is a normal process. It's not always the same as depression. Sometimes, you have to go through it to get to the other side.

- Sometimes, when you lose something so close to you, you feel the need to show it through changing a part of your identity too. And that's okay. You feel different on the inside, so changing on the outside feels natural.

- The relationships in your life will probably be impacted by your loss. Sometimes, that might not always be a bad thing. Some might change for the better. Others might not. These might be hard lessons to learn.

- Even though you very much want your partner to understand what you are going through, be prepared for the fact that they might not. Everyone grieves differently.

- Not everyone will know what to say. Some people will say things that are hurtful. Some people will won't say anything at all, and that might feel worse. And some people will say things that are just beautiful.

- When you are ready to have another child that doesn't mean that you will have forgotten about the baby you've lost. When you're feeling a little better it doesn't mean that you are "moving on." It just means that you are finding new strength and that your grief has changed.

Finding support

Women discover different ways of finding support and what works for you might not work for someone else. Some women are very blessed to have extremely communicative partners while others have difficulty expressing difficult emotions with theirs and instead find their support in online forums. Some good places to find support include:

- Hospital prenatal loss groups

- Hospice centers

- Online pregnancy loss groups

- Pregnancy centers

- Counseling centers

- Community centers

- Your doctor's office

Counseling can be a very good way of finding an unbiased ear. However, keep in mind that counseling's benefits are long-term and aren't a quick fix. Although the benefits of counseling will come to you eventually, they will take time. You may have to wait for your appointment to come. If you need someone to talk to right away, this can be difficult.

Support groups can help fill in those gaps. Counselors, especially grief counselors, are trained to help you understand your feelings and emotions and put them in perspective and in context to your experience. Over time, that's very helpful. In a support group, whether you find that online or offline, you'll meet people who are going through a similar experience and you can reach out to those people any time-day or night. Communicating with others who have experienced a similar loss can ease some of the isolation, and help to make sense of how you're feeling.

Some popular online support groups for ectopic pregnancy losses include:

- Ectopic Pregnancy: Baby Center: New Hopes: http://community.babycenter.com/groups/a734235/ectopic_pregnancy_-_new_hopes

- Ectopic Pregnancy & Miscarriage Support: Café Mom: http://www.cafemom.com/group/23916

- Ectopic Pregnancy Trust: http://www.ectopic.org.uk/talk/

- Baby Centre Community: http://community.babycentre.co.uk/

Grieving

An ectopic pregnancy can have a huge emotional impact on you and those around you, including your partner and even your parents. The grief process from an ectopic pregnancy varies slightly from other forms of pregnancy loss. Not only are you are grieving the loss of your baby and dealing with the emotional aspect of the loss of pregnancy, if you had surgery you're also trying to recuperate from that as well. It can be difficult to balance the two.

Some women also struggle with the idea that the budding embryo may have also been developing normally and even had a heartbeat at the time of the surgery, although this is very, very rare. You may logically know that the baby couldn't have grown to term, but it's natural to have mixed feelings about having to terminate the pregnancy.

Well meaning people can make comments that are meant to be helpful but can be unintentionally hurtful or callous in the process. You might hear comments that minimize your loss, like "At least you weren't pregnant long." Even though it was an early pregnancy loss doesn't mean you're still not grieving the loss.

Not only can grief have an emotional impact on your mental health, it can have physical symptoms, too. Some of the physical symptoms of grief include:

• fatigue

• loss of appetite

• trouble concentrating

• difficulty sleeping

Emotional symptoms of grief include:

• guilt

• numbness

• anger

- an overwhelming sense of sadness

Symptoms are usually worse 4-6 weeks after the loss of pregnancy before slowly improving. However, it can take as long as a full year (or even longer) before some women start to fully feel like themselves again. The feelings of sadness may never really go away, but grief can change and adapt over time and this can make moving forward easier.

Even though the grief that follows an ectopic pregnancy can feel unbearable at times, it's actually a type of healing process. Denying grief and the feelings that accompany it can actually suppress the process and make things harder on your physical and emotional health. This can make the healing process last far longer so, as far as you're able, it's helpful to allow yourselves to feel the emotional pain that inevitably comes with an ectopic pregnancy.

Talking to your partner

Partners often find it hard to understand your feelings, simply because they didn't have the physical attachment to the pregnancy that you did and didn't go through the physical and emotional symptoms of the pregnancy. You might sometimes feel as though your partner doesn't care or isn't as supportive of you as you feel he should be. Sometimes, you might feel ignored. If you've gone through surgery, you might be suffering from the aftermath of treatment and be unable to participate in physical activities that you used to enjoy and this may make you feel depressed which could compound your frustrations.

Communication is always vital in any relationship but it's especially important after the loss of a pregnancy. Unfortunately, sometimes there is a breakdown of communication just at the point when it should be strongest. This isn't anyone's fault, but often both partners are so focused on trying to sort out their own feelings and emotions that they're really unsure on how to care for the other person. Men, too, often want to "fix" things and sometimes have trouble understanding that in this particular situation the there isn't anything to be "fixed" and they don't know what to do with that.

As a way to make you feel "better" your partner might try to distract you by buying you things, changing the subject, or even avoid talking about the pregnancy loss. This might make you feel even worse, as though your partner doesn't care about the fact that the two of you lost a baby. However, you must realize that he isn't doing this because he doesn't care - this is simply his way of attempting to deal with the experience and cope in his own way. Talking about your feelings and communicating will help break down these barriers.

Helping each other through the loss

Go slowly

Try to take your time. There is no deadline for grief and you can't rush it. If you set a clock on your partner and try to push him to keep pace with your own feelings and emotions then things could get bad quickly. You should both try to work at your own speed, both in emotionally and physically. You'll both have good days and bad days. Hopefully, some of those good days will fall on the same day from time to time and eventually that will happen more and more.

Be respectful

Understand the fact that you both have different ways of grieving and then respect that. There is no right or wrong way to grieve. Simply treating one another with respect will go a long way in helping one another. By extending the freedom to grieve in the way that works for them, you're allowing your partner to do what feels right. This allows for honesty and communication in your relationship.

Do things together

Even though you might want to grieve in private, it's still important to do things as a couple. Just getting out on occasion and remembering why you're together in the first place is helpful. Going for a walk around the neighborhood, seeing a movie, and spending time together can be healing. You don't you have to do anything expensive or extravagant, but often the partner can feel neglected and couples time can be good for the soul.

Honor the loss

Honoring the pregnancy in a way that's reflective is a good way to bring the two of you together and talk about your feelings. It doesn't have to be anything big, but it can open up the lines of communication and help you talk about your loss. However, you might want to refrain from doing this continuously. This is something you might want to do once, or do on an anniversary. If all of your "couples time" revolves around your loss then it might keep you from moving forward in your grief and this could be detrimental to your grieving process.

If you're concerned that you and your partner are having difficulties coping with grief or communicating with one another it's possible that you might need help from an unbiased third party. It is generally not recommended that you seek help from a friend or family member since that can put that person in an awkward position and make them feel like they must chose sides. Instead, you might want to consider joining a support group or attending counseling sessions where the two of you can talk to other couples who have gone through a similar loss or talk to an impartial mediator.

Chapter 7: Recovering from the physical strain

Your body has been through a traumatic course of events and it's going to be a little while before it recovers. Whether you have surgery, take the Methotrexate, or let your body absorb the pregnancy, it will still take time to adjust and heal. It's important that you take it easy on yourself and remember to be gentle with your body as well as with your heart.

Recovering from surgery

How long you will stay in the hospital will depend on the type of surgery you had. For a laparoscopy, some women have out-patient procedures. Others stay 1-2 days. For a laparotomy, the average stay is 2-3 days. For abdominal surgeries, the average stay is 3-4 days.

After a surgery, most women experience pain during the first 1-2 weeks, depending on the type of surgery they had. For a laparoscopy, the recovery time is significantly shorter than abdominal surgery. Some women are able to get up and walk around with relative ease later that day; in fact, most doctors want their patients up moving around a little bit that evening. Not only does it help relieve constipation but it can help patients avoid blood clots and bed sores. A change of scenery can be good for the soul after lying in bed all day. You don't want to overdo it, but getting up and moving from the bed to the sofa can be a nice change.

The doctor will more than likely prescribe you pain pills and these can make you feel a little loopy at first. You might also feel nauseated and dizzy and maybe even sick for the first couple of days. If you have had a laparoscopy then you might also feel bloated and may even feel pain in your stomach from the trapped gas. Some women find that the pain is more severe upon sitting up. The pain gets better as time goes by and is alleviated with the pain mediation and from walking around. If constipation is an issue then you can buy many natural and gentle laxatives which can help ease this problem. It's really important to drink plenty of water.

For the first day or two you might not feel like eating much. That is okay. Focus on drinking fluids and eating light meals. On the other hand, you might be very hungry. Just try to listen to what your body wants. If you're nauseated then stick to bland foods, such as rice and crackers, and don't eat anything too greasy or heavy.

You might also feel very tired as your body recovers not only from the pregnancy, but also from the surgery. Get as much rest as possible since sleep is when your body will repair itself. If you lost any blood then you may have also had a blood transfusion while you were in the hospital. Your doctor may have sent iron tablets home with you to help increase your iron if you still have signs of anemia. Continue taking these because one of the major symptoms of anemia is fatigue. You'll need your energy up to start feeling yourself again.

Many hospitals ask for a follow-up appointment in about 6 weeks and some hospitals will call and check on you to see how you're doing. A laparoscopy is generally an out-patient procedure but if you had a lot of vomiting or pain you might have to spend a night before being released. If you have hypertension or any other underlying medical conditions that need extra care and observation then these might also require you to spend extra time in the hospital.

Your own doctor will want to see you back in his office in around 6 weeks in any case, just to check on you and see how your stitches are healing. These days, most stitches that are used dissolve on their own. Others are simply removed painlessly with a pair of tweezers in your doctor's office at the follow-up appointment.

Before your follow-up appointment, however, you will probably still return to your doctor to have your hCG levels checked, just to ensure that they are dropping the way that they should be.

If you had abdominal surgery then your recovery will be longer and you'll spend more time in the hospital. Abdominal surgery is somewhat more painful and can have more risks involved. The recovery time can take anywhere from 6-8 weeks. During that time, it's important not to lift anything heavier than 5 pounds. Your doctor will still probably want you up walking around within 24 hours, however, and trying to move as much as possible without exerting yourself.

In many cases, you may be advised not to drive for a certain period of time, at least whilst you are on strong pain medication. Still, regardless of which surgery you had, continue to take any pain medication as prescribed. Staying on schedule with this will help aid in your recovery as many pain medications loose some of their effectiveness if doses are missed.

Questions to ask

At your follow-up appointment, you might ask some of the following questions:

- Was there any obvious reason why I had the ectopic pregnancy?

- Was there any damage to the fallopian tubes?

- Was there any evidence of scar tissue or adhesions anywhere else in my abdomen?

- (If you had your tube removed or repaired) Did my remaining tube look healthy and okay?

- When can I start trying to conceive again?

- When will I need to come back here?

- If I become pregnant again, what kind of support or early pregnancy screening will be available to me in this office?

Tips to help in your recovery

- Keep the incision clean. When you bathe, keep it dry and away from the water. If you go outside, ensure you keep it clean until the stitches have been removed and the skin has closed up.

- Get plenty of rest but also walk around a little bit every day. Take walks around your house and around your garden or local park if you can manage it. Try to increase your distance a little every day. Avoid stairs for the first week if you've had abdominal surgery.

- If your bedroom is upstairs, consider making a bed on the couch or in a spare bedroom downstairs so that you don't have to climb the stairs, which could be hard on your stitches.

- Avoid any heavy lifting for about 2 weeks.

- Forget about housework and chores for a couple of weeks. It will all be there later.

- Keep to gentle exercise like walking. Once your wound has healed, add swimming to your exercises since it gently stretches your muscles.

- Bath and shower regularly, but keep your wound dry. Unless your nurse tells you otherwise, you can shower 24-48 hours after surgery. If you do take a bath or shower, though, have someone nearby, especially if you still feel faint or dizzy.

- Have your nurse talk to you about pelvic floor exercises, called Kegel exercises, which can help strengthen your pelvic floor. This can greatly help increase your muscles which is of benefit to both your bladder and vagina.

- Take your pain medication as prescribed. If it helps create a time chart or set a phone alarm or give them to a partner or someone who lives with you and have them schedule them for you so that you don't have to remember when to take them. Don't wait until you're in pain to take them since they're not as effective that way.

- Have someone else prepare meals ahead of time and come in and help you so that you don't have to worry about cooking.

- If you have little children at home, ask a family member or friend to watch them for a couple of days while you recover. The first few days are the hardest and an extra set of eyes and help can be valuable, especially where little ones are concerned.

Recovering from Methotrexate

Methotrexate has its own set of recovery challenges, but they're not unlike those of surgery. Many women find themselves feeling exhausted, sluggish, and even a little depressed. Doctors advise women not to start exercising until their hCG levels drop to the low 100's, although once you are able to start being active again you'll probably find that your energy levels do start picking back up.

Unlike with surgery, driving isn't prohibited after medical treatment with Methotrexate. If you feel like you're having trouble managing your emotions or you're having difficulty with grief or depression you might want to talk to your doctor before you operate a car.

Grief and depression is nothing to feel ashamed about and many women do find that immediately following treatment of an ectopic pregnancy they are dealing with emotions they've never experienced before. In addition, there might also still be some symptoms present such as light-headedness and dizziness so ensure that you feel comfortable and safe driving before you embark on any road adventures.

When it comes to returning to work, women who were treated with Methotrexate sometimes work while going through the treatment but others find it too difficult, especially if they are symptomatic. In most cases, you should be able to return to work within 4-6 weeks. Some women do take off longer, however, whilst others want to work so they can focus on something else for a time. This will depend on how you are feeling physically and emotionally, and what your company's work policy is. It may be a good idea to do a detox, even if it's just a mild one, following treatment with Methotrexate though you'll want to wait until a month or so when your body has recovered somewhat – we discuss tips for detoxing later.

Chapter 8: Subsequent Pregnancies

Many women who have experienced one ectopic pregnancy do go on to have successful, subsequent, intrauterine pregnancies.

Of the women who do not have an intrauterine pregnancy after having an ectopic one, in some cases it is because they simply do not wish to conceive again. In other cases, it is because they suffer from infertility (for different reasons) and are unable to conceive. In addition, there is also the fact that having a previous ectopic pregnancy does increase the risk of having a subsequent one. However, with advancements in technology and more research, it is hopeful that statistics will keep improving and that more and more subsequent pregnancies will be viable, intrauterine ones.

The success rates of the subsequent pregnancies are somewhat determined by how early the preceding ectopic pregnancy was discovered. In addition, it's also important to note whether or not any damage was done to the fallopian tubes, particularly if any scar tissue developed within the tubes that might make it difficult for the transport of sperm and egg to get to where they need to travel.

For those women who have had a fallopian tube removed, it's still possible to conceive. As long as you have one healthy tube functioning, you can still get pregnant.

However, if the previous ectopic pregnancy was due to damage to the tube because of tubal ligation or an infection such as PID, then there is still a chance that the existing fallopian tube is also damaged. This can not only make conceiving more difficult, but will make the likelihood of having another ectopic pregnancy stronger.

Fertility after an ectopic pregnancy

While the chances of having a successful pregnancy after an ectopic pregnancy may be somewhat lower than normal for most women, they will depend on why the pregnancy was ectopic as well as your medical history. The chances of going on and having a future successful pregnancy after experiencing an ectopic pregnancy in the past depend in part on:

- Whether or not you've successfully given birth in the past

- Your age

- The cause of the last ectopic pregnancy

- The state of the fallopian tubes

Try to keep in mind that statistically chances are you will achieve a successful pregnancy in the future. Even if you have other factors acting against you, remember that thousands of people get pregnant and have healthy babies against far more unlikely odds every year, so as hard as it may feel at times, do try and stay positive.

Salpingectomy by laparotomy has a subsequent intrauterine pregnancy rate of 25-70%, compared with laparoscopic salpingectomy rates of 50-60%. The rates for laparoscopic salpingotomy versus laparotomy are similar. When a huge range for success occurs, such as with a salpingectomy by laparotomy, it can feel pretty unhelpful. It's definitely worth talking to your doctor about your specific circumstances whilst again trying not to focus too much on any worrying statistics.

Remember that before you start trying to conceive ovulation will actually occur *before* your period. You can even ovulate within 14 days after. Even if you've had one or both of your fallopian tubes removed, you'll still have a period. The fallopian tubes don't have anything to do with your menstrual cycle. The menstrual cycle is controlled by hormones that are mostly located within the ovaries.

When to try again

Many women are excited to try to conceive again after losing a pregnancy. After all, they found out they were pregnant, only to turn around (sometimes in the same week) to discover that the pregnancy was not a viable one. It's a heartbreaking experience and the grief is one that can last a lifetime. Still, the timing of the subsequent pregnancy is a crucial one and it's important to take several factors into consideration, not just for your own health, but for your future child's as well.

Most doctors recommend that you wait at least two full cycles before trying to conceive again, but most would prefer that you wait three and maybe even up to six months. A three month wait not only gives your body the chance to heal, but depending on the form of treatment that was used for the ectopic pregnancy, it can be dangerous to the developing fetus to try too soon.

The first time that you bleed after experiencing an ectopic pregnancy is not a true menstrual cycle; this is merely the bleeding that occurs in response to the falling hormones associated with the loss of the pregnancy. It could also be in response to the treatment option that you were given.

By waiting at least two or three cycles, you are allowing your cycles to get back to normal. This will also allow you to plan more clearly for a plain LMP (last menstrual period) date, which will allow you to date a new pregnancy. In addition, by waiting several cycles, your body will have time to heal from any surgeries you had and the internal inflammation will be able to heal as well. This is especially important if you had any work done on your fallopian tubes.

For those who have been treated with Methotrexate, waiting at least three months is crucial since it probably reduced the level of folate in your body. Folate deficiencies could cause neural tube defects in the baby, such as spina bifida. Most doctors recommend that you start taking folic acid for at least a month before you start trying to conceive; however, you can't start taking folic acid until your hCG levels are below 5<mIU/mL. Since folic acid helps build strong, healthy babies by assisting with cell division, and you're essentially trying to keep that

from happening when you're treating an ectopic pregnancy, folic acid will be counterproductive to the process.

After your blood hCG levels have dropped, if you want to start trying to conceive, you should continue your folic acid supplements several weeks or months before you start trying to become pregnant again.

hCG tests

It is important that your hCG levels are rechecked on a regular basis until they reach zero if your entire fallopian tube wasn't removed. If you have hCG levels that remain high, it could indicate that the ectopic tissue wasn't completely removed. This might mean that surgery is necessary or, if you only had a single dose of Methotrexate, that an additional dose is necessary. If your doctor was using expectant management then rising levels would mean that medical intervention would be needed, either in the form of medication or surgery.

Subsequent pregnancy management

When you find out you're pregnant, you should alert your healthcare provider as soon as possible. Your doctor will probably want to perform an early ultrasound at around 6 or 7 weeks to ensure that the implantation is within the uterus. Since you are considered high risk in the early stages, you will be monitored more closely at the beginning of your pregnancy.

Blood work may be carried out several times to ensure that your hCG levels are rising as normal. It will be important to document any symptoms and to alert your doctor if you have any abdominal cramping, dizziness, light-headedness, fainting, shoulder pain, or vaginal bleeding.

Once it is confirmed that the pregnancy is intrauterine and not ectopic then your doctor will talk to you about continuing the pregnancy on a more standard schedule with regular appointments. Repeated blood work, at this point, will not be as necessary since the biggest worry is at the beginning when the question is where the developing egg sac is located.

Chances of reoccurrence

More than 85% of all ectopic pregnancies are discovered in the first trimester (LL Marion, 2012). Most of is this due to advancements in the medical field such as transvaginal ultrasounds and blood tests that can detect hCG levels. As a result, laparoscopic surgery has led to tubal preservation, which has been able to preserve tubal fertility.

The chances of having another ectopic pregnancy are around 10-20%.

Can I prevent another one?

Unfortunately, there really isn't anything anyone can do to prevent an ectopic pregnancy. However, if you think that your history of pelvic infections caused by STIs (particularly Chlamydia trachomatis) caused your last ectopic pregnancy then getting testing and antibiotic treatment for this might reduce the risk of a future ectopic pregnancy.

Some women do undergo surgery to have adhesions removed. There is a possibility that the removal of adhesions can potentially improve the possibility of conceiving, especially if you're having fertility issues. This surgery is generally referred to as a hysteroscopy for the removal of adhesions or scar tissue, if it is being done inside the uterus, or a simple laparoscopy if it's outside the uterus. Not only can it help improve fertility chances, it can also help relieve pain, especially if adhesions have caused parts of the wall of the uterus or even other organs to stick together, or if you have another underlying medical condition such as endometriosis or adenomyosis.

However, adhesions may come back after they have been removed and scar tissue can form post surgery as well so it's generally advised that you start trying to conceive as soon as possible. Though there is evidence that many couples have had successful pregnancies after this type of surgery, some doctors do advise against having adhesions removed since it is estimated that in some cases, the surgery to remove the original adhesions could cause even more to develop. You should discuss the risks and benefits thoroughly with your healthcare provider so

that you can make an informed decision about what's right
for you.

Chapter 9: Conceiving again

After having such a heartbreaking and scary experience, not every woman wishes to conceive again, but many women are anxious to try to have another baby - and as soon as they can. If you've been trying for at least six months and are having difficulty conceiving, then you might be thinking about fertility treatments. You might also be wondering if your previous experience has hindered your chances at conceiving again. The good news is, your chances really haven't been hurt as much as you might think, and even though some fertility treatments might slightly increase risks of a subsequent ectopic pregnancy, they're not as high as you may fear.

Keeping track of cycles

It might sound obvious but keeping track of your menstrual cycles is one of the most important things you can do when you're trying to conceive again. Although most doctors recommend having regular sexual intercourse throughout your cycle for your best chances of conceiving, by keeping track of your cycles you'll be able to plan your intercourse around your days that are most fertile. You can do this by several ways, either by purchasing ovulation kits, as we'll discuss in a moment, or by keeping a calendar and learning the pattern of your cycles yourself.

Although the obvious signs and symptoms of your monthly cycle is the bleeding that comes with your period, there are actually other signs to watch out for as well.

During ovulation, there are hormonal changes that take place and these can cause physical symptoms. When you pay attention to your body and learn these symptoms, you can sometimes tell when you're most fertile and close to ovulating.

5 Signs of Ovulation

1. Egg white mucous: It doesn't sound nice, but when your cervical mucous (which you can often see as a discharge if you watch out for it) turns the color and consistency of egg whites, that's when it's best for transporting sperm.

2. You feel more lubricated: If you notice that you just feel a little wetter in your vaginal area and that you're more naturally lubricated during intercourse, then you might be close to ovulating. This is nature's way of preparing your body to accept sperm.

3. Sore breasts: During ovulation, and right after it, progesterone levels can rise. This can cause breast tenderness.

4. Slight cramping: Some women have slight cramping during ovulation. This pain has a name and it's called mittelschmerz. It might be caused by the egg breaking through the follicle or as the

fallopian tube narrows to move the egg into the uterus.

5. Migraines: Hormones during ovulation trigger migraines in about 20% of women. If you suffer from these headaches then chances are, you are entering your peak fertile period.

There are some websites out there that can help you chart your cycle for free. My Monthly Cycles, for instance, (http://mymonthlycycles.com/) offers a wealth of information including tools that will help you track your most fertile days, your next period, symptoms of fertility, and expected due date.

Fertility treatments

For some women who have damaged fallopian tubes, fertility treatments like in vitro fertilization (IVF) might be a good option. There are other treatment options available, too, to help women have successful pregnancies after experiencing an ectopic one. This is something you might want to discuss with your healthcare provider if you have tried to conceive again after experiencing an ectopic pregnancy and have been unable to get pregnant.

Clomid

Clomiphene, or Clomid, is a powerful medication that is often prescribed for women who have trouble with infertility. It's also one of the first courses of action if a woman is having difficulty conceiving since it's a tablet that can be prescribed in a doctor's office and doesn't require any injections.

Clomid blocks the hormone estrogen receptors in your brain. In the beginning of your cycle, your estrogen levels are low. Most of the time, the eggs will mature and they'll produce estrogen. These levels will increase as the eggs mature and eventually the estrogen levels will tell the body to produce the luteinizing hormone. This is what will cause ovulation to take place.

Clomid is not that different from estrogen in its chemical makeup. Your brain has a hard time telling the difference and this lets it attach to your brain's receptor cells. However, when Clomid attaches to the cells, your own estrogen is unable to. As a result, the body believes you're not making adequate estrogen. Consequently, your body starts making other hormones that help cultivate the follicles within the ovaries (which is good for enhanced fertility) since these are what produce estrogen and your body wants those levels to increase.

The recommended dose for the first course is 50mg (1 tablet) daily for 5 days. It can be started at any time as long as there hasn't been any recent uterine bleeding. If there hasn't been any ovulation after the first course of therapy, a second course of 100mg daily for 5 days can be given. This course can be started 30 days after the last one. Some women conceive after the first course of therapy, and more conceive after the second. A third can be given, but if by the third, you still haven't fallen pregnant then the doctor will usually look for other reasons why you haven't conceived and consider other options. Clomid is not given to women who have ovarian cysts.

Clomid does have the reputation for occasionally working so well that it supplies a woman with not one baby but two. Although there are not any statistics to support the number of cases this happens in, Clomid can increase the chances of having twins since it can basically encourage your body to produce more than one egg by increasing your estrogen levels. If your body releases more than one egg during ovulation and both of these are fertilized then twins are the result of this action. Of course, this doesn't always happen, but it can.

It is important to remember that there is an increased chance of ectopic pregnancy (including tubal and ovarian sites) in those who conceive following Clomid 50mg therapy. Multiple pregnancies, including simultaneous intrauterine and extrauterine pregnancies, have been reported using this kind of fertility treatment. The rate is low, less than 1%, depending on the source, but it still exists. Of course, there is also a chance that you might end up pregnant with multiple babies as well since that occurs more frequently, too.

Intrauterine Insemination (IUI)

Some women end up utilizing intrauterine insemination (IUI). Also known as "artificial insemination", this is a procedure in which "cleaned" sperm is placed inside a uterus for fertilization. The goal of this is to boost the number of sperm that reach the fallopian tubes. As part of the process, hCG is administered to encourage the release of eggs from the follicles. An advantage of this procedure is that it doesn't involve manipulating the woman's eggs, and therefore it isn't considered an assisted reproductive technology (ART) procedure. This last fact may make it a good choice for anyone who's religion may not support assisted reproductive technology methods, or who just don't feel personally comfortable with them.

IUI is most often used when a couple has been trying to conceive for at least a year. It's also commonly used by couples where maternal age is a factor or who are experiencing unexplained infertility. For women with a history of ectopic pregnancy, it might be a consideration since it can be used when there is cervical scar tissue present from past surgical procedures or adhesions from conditions such as endometriosis. It might also prove useful following a surgery to remove scar tissue as it could help pregnancy occur quickly - before any new scars have the chance to form.

The average success rate for IUI is about 10-20% in one cycle, with women under the age of 35 being the most successful. IUI will normally be tried for 3-4 cycles as the success rates can be cumulative with rates being at around 20-33% for 4-6 cycles.

An ovulation predictor kit, and sometimes transvaginal ultrasounds will help determine which days are most fertile so that the doctor can insert the sperm at the optimal time.

Sometimes IUI is combined with injectable drugs to stimulate the ovaries and ensure egg production and timed release.

IVF treatments

In IVF treatments, a fertilized egg that has reached the Zygote stage (the cells have started dividing) is placed in the uterus from 1-2 days after fertilization or from to 4-5 days from when it has developed many more cells and is referred to as a blastocyst. IVF treatment has a high success rate of pregnancy, but it also has a risk of ectopic pregnancy (1-3%) since the egg can have several days of floating around before it implants. It is possible for the egg to float into a tube or into the interstitial area of the uterus and implant there.

hCG trigger shot

Some women who have been trying to conceive for several months and have been unsuccessful find success with the hCG trigger shot, although not all medical clinics offer this option. This shot contains a synthetic form of the hormone human chorionic gonadotropin. Brand names include Ovidrel, Profasi, Pregnyl, and Novarel.

Known as the "pregnancy hormone" and important during ectopic pregnancies, hCG maintains the corpus luteum which is in charge of progesterone production during the second half of the menstrual cycle and in early pregnancy.

Before taking the shot, you would most likely be given a medication such as Clomid first. This will help your ovaries develop follicles that are necessary for ovulation. The shot can then help ensure that the mature eggs are released from the follicles.

If you and your doctor decide this is the best option for you, you will be closely monitored. Ultrasounds will be used to observe the progress of the developing follicles to determine if the eggs are preparing to be released. When the follicles are mature, instructions will be given on how to take the trigger shot, which is something you can actually do yourself. It sounds, and even looks a little scary but really doesn't hurt more than a little pinch and many needle-phobic women have successfully managed to either self administer the shot – or persuade a helpful partner to do it for them.

Not long after taking the trigger shot, usually within 36 hours, you should get a positive ovulation test. This will tell you that you've reached a peak fertile period and that you are ovulating. Some clinics will combine the trigger shot and IUI for an additional fertility boost.

Low progesterone

Some women find that they have trouble conceiving, or maintaining an early pregnancy because they suffer from low progesterone. The hormone progesterone is responsible for several things within the body that must take place in order for a healthy pregnancy to happen and be maintained.

The pituitary gland in the brain fuels the ovaries to secrete estrogen and progesterone at different times. Progesterone is particularly important since it is responsible for making sure the lining of the uterus is ready for implantation. It is also responsible for maintaining a pregnancy. After ovulation, progesterone is secreted from the ovary by a tissue called a "corpus luteum." This is maintained by the hCG until the placenta can take over the production of progesterone. If pregnancy doesn't occur, the corpus luteum will expire, progesterone levels plunge and the menstrual cycle will start all over again.

Low progesterone symptoms:

Sometimes, low progesterone symptoms will imitate other disorders so it's hard to tell that you have anything wrong. Infertility and pregnancy loss is often the only thing that happens to make your doctor look into your progesterone levels. However, there are other symptoms to be on the lookout for.

Low progesterone symptoms can include:

- Depression
- Insomnia
- Sugar cravings
- Ovarian cysts

- Changes in appetite
- Weight fluctuations
- Irritability
- Inability to concentrate
- Anxiety
- Fatigue
- Irregular menstruation
- Low sex drive
- Migraines
- PCOS (Polycystic Ovarian Syndrome)
- Vaginal dryness
- Frequent menstruation
- Painful intercourse

Causes of low progesterone:

Sometimes, the cause of low progesterone levels is unknown. Sometimes, a woman might not have any difficulty getting pregnant but the placenta doesn't create the proper levels of progesterone when it should. Some things that might contribute to low levels of progesterone include lack of exercise, high levels of stress, and poor nutrition.

Boosting progesterone levels

If you or your doctor suspects low progesterone levels he or she will need to carry out some blood work to see if this is an issue.

If low progesterone is confirmed there are progesterone supplements (Prometrium being one of the most popular) that can be taken right before you ovulate and then for the second part of your menstrual cycle, or even longer if you do fall pregnant. Some are taken in tablet form while others are taken as suppositories. There are also progesterone creams, which have been used with limited success when it comes to trying to conceive (the prescriptions have had more success with the creams coming in a close second). Progesterone supplements can help with implantation and with maintaining a pregnancy. There are also natural ways of boosting progesterone levels as well.

The HSG test

If you have tried to conceive for at least 6 months and are over the age of 35, you might consider getting the HSG test. The Hysterosalpingogram test (HSG) is only usually performed after a period of trying to conceive without success, and the majority of doctors won't even consider it until you've been trying to conceive for at least a year. The reason is that there is a small risk of infection, which may outweigh the benefits so it's important to discuss this risk with your doctor.

A HSG test requires an X-ray to look at the interior of the uterus and fallopian tubes to see if anything is going on in them to determine why you're unable to conceive. During the test, a dye is inserted using a thin tube through the vagina and into the uterus. Pictures are taken as the dye passes through the tubes and uterus.

The images will show any issues such as blockages, injuries, adhesions, or abnormal structures that might prevent the egg from moving through the fallopian tubes. A blockage could keep the sperm from being able to move through the tube and fertilizing the egg. A HSG test can also look for issues inside the uterus that might keep a fertilized egg from implanting such as adhesions, polyps, or fibroids.

Before the test starts, the doctor will usually administer a soft sedative that will relax you and your uterus so that it won't cramp and spasm during the test. You'll remove your clothes below the waist and put on a hospital gown and empty your bladder. You'll lie on your back and place your feet in stirrups. A curved speculum is placed into the vagina, similar to pelvic exams, to open the vaginal walls and allow the doctor to look into the cervix. The cervix is then washed with a special kind of soap and a catheter is inserted through the cervix into the uterus. The X-ray dye is put through the tube. This is important since if the fallopian tubes are open, the dye will go through them and spill into the stomach. If the fallopian tubes are blocked, the dye won't go through them and that gives doctors another way of determining if there is a problem.

When the test is completed, usually in about 15 minutes, the catheter and speculum are removed. Most women find that there is some pressure and mild discomfort, but the test isn't painful for most women.

Some women do find that the test itself can help them get pregnant as the process can even help unwind small kinks in the fallopian tube and potentially remove mucous or even small scar tissues.

Having only one tube left

Even when you only have one remaining tube, it's still highly possible to get pregnant. Both ovaries are usually left, unless there has been damage to the ovaries as well. In that case, generally at least one ovary is left behind. Every month, the ovaries compete with one another to produce an egg. The one that produces an egg first is the one that "wins" while the other one "gives up" in most cases.

During ovulation, even though the egg usually travels down the fallopian tube it's closest to, that doesn't always happen. Even if you have a tube removed that doesn't necessarily mean that your chances of conceiving will be limited. When you ovulate, the fimbriae will move and gently create a small vacuum motion to suck the egg toward the end of the tube it is closest to. If there is only one tube then there's only one set of fimbriae to create a vacuum and the egg is more inclined to travel to that tube, regardless of which ovary produced it.

If an egg is produced on the side that doesn't have a fallopian tube then it will still normally find its way to the side that does have a tube about 15 to 20% of the time.

As a result, your fertility isn't even cut in half, it's only slightly reduced.

Ovulation Predictor Kits (OPK)

Ovulation predictor kits (OPKs) are valuable since they can help you to discover your fertile window. While, having intercourse regularly is the best way to maximize your chances of conceiving, you may prefer to concentrate sex during your fertile period if either one of you are away from home a lot and it makes regular intercourse challenging or if you have busy schedules. If you're subject to irregular cycles then an OPK can also be helpful in determining when your most fertile period is.

An OPK can be purchased at most pharmacists, as well as online, and it lets you identify your fertile window from the first month. The urine-based tests measure your urine for a surge in the luteinizing hormone (LH) which occurs 1-2 days before ovulation. There is always a little bit of this in your blood and urine but right before ovulation, it increases. In the 12-36 hours between the beginning of the LH surge and before your egg is released is when you're most fertile.

The salivary ferning kits let you test your saliva with a small microscope. When your estrogen levels rise, the salt in your salvia rises, too. When the salt dries up, it crystallizes into a pattern that looks like a fern. (Hence the name.) This is more likely to happen right before you ovulate.

The salivary tests are sometimes easier to handle and not as messy, but they're also not as accurate. Some people have trouble deciphering the patterns. They are meant to be used first thing in the morning, before you've had anything to eat or drink.

Popular OPKs

- **First Response Easy Read Ovulation Test** US $19.39 The First Response Easy-Read Ovulation Test is over 99% accurate in laboratory studies. It detects the luteinizing hormone (LH) surge in the urine and therefore indicates when you're most fertile. The kit contains 7 testing sticks, one for each day of the week.

- **Fertile Focus** US $27.95 Fertile Focus is a saliva-based fertility test that predicts ovulation with 98% accuracy up to 72 hours in advance.

  http://www.fairhavenhealth.com/fertile-focus.html

- **Clearblue Easy Digital Ovulation Test** UK £32.78 US $36 Identifies your four best days to conceive. It comes with 20 sticks, or a 2 month supply. A smiley face appears on your peak fertility days.

- **True Ultra Sensitive Ovulation Test Strips (30 pack)** UK £10.00. Detects the LH surge at 20miu/ml and indicates the 2 most fertile days of your cycle.

- It is over 99.5% accurate and has easy to read results.

Chapter 10: Boosting Fertility

Most women don't immediately start off by turning to expensive fertility treatments, some of which can be invasive. Instead, they like to try natural methods of boosting their fertility. Considering that as many as 85% of women conceive within the first 18 months after an ectopic pregnancy (when they're trying to conceive) following some of the practices below might be a good step in the right direction when it comes to preparing your body for your next pregnancy and making it primed and ready.

Regular Sex

During your fertile period, most fertility experts recommend you try to have intercourse at least every two days. This will increase the amount of sperm that is released during intercourse, especially if your partner has an issue with low sperm count. Most women ovulate between days 12-16 of their cycles and their luteal phase is around 10-12 days long. The luteal phase begins on the day you start ovulating and stops the day before your next period begins.

Not only is it important to have intercourse when you are ovulating, it can help to engage in intercourse before your luteal phase starts, too. The egg will survive for about 1-3 days once it is released. However, sperm can survive for as long as a week. As a result, there is actually up to a six-day window for healthy sperm to meet an egg and fertilize it.

The intercourse you have before you're fertile period begins may boost your chances of getting good swimming sperm when you need it. Even after ovulation occurs, regular sex may improve your chances of getting pregnant since semen may play a part in embryo development and implantation, although there haven't been many studies done on this yet.

The position you choose might also play a part in your chances of conception. The missionary position (the woman lying on her back with her pelvis tilted upwards) allows the sperm to enter the cervix and into the uterus at the optimal angle. Some women swear by resting on their backs with their legs gently raised slightly by a pillow and relaxing in this position for about 15-20 minutes after sex and there is some evidence that indicates this may increase your chances of conception so it's worth a try if and when that's possible.

Don't ignore your vaginal health

The environment within your vagina should be friendly to sperm and welcoming. This means avoiding any kind to sprays, scents, or douches. If you use tampons during your menstrual cycle, only use only 100% organic cotton tampons. If you take antibiotics and subsequently get a yeast infection, take a really good acidophilus and probiotic supplement which can add the "healthy" bacteria back into your body and put your digestive system back on track.

Studies have found that a lot of lubricants are harmful to sperm (Anderson L, 1998). Popular lubricants can inhibit sperm movement and even kill sperm (Kutteh WH, 1996) so they're best avoided for optimum fertility.

There are some lubricants that are designed for couples who have trouble with lubrication. Pre-Seed, for example, is vagina and conception friendly.

Increase Your Fertile Mucous

Cervical mucous is important because it transports sperm and eggs. It shouldn't be too thick. In fact, during your fertile period, it should be the consistency of egg whites. Some women, however, have trouble producing cervical mucous and others have trouble producing the right consistency. This can inhibit the transportation of sperm to the egg. Not having any cervical mucous can be called "hostile cervical mucous" and this can cause infertility.

A healthy diet can increase the production of fertile cervical mucous. Try to avoid eating excessive amounts of dairy and wheat products since these can make the vaginal mucus too thick. Hydration is important, especially purified water, since this can help give the cervical mucous the watery consistency it needs.

Some women also find that they have more abundant fertile cervical mucous when they drink a large glass of grapefruit juice every day during the last week before ovulation. Grapefruit juice can improve the consistency of the mucous and make it thinner. Even though it is acidic, after it's digested it has an alkalizing effect and this can help make the mucus even friendlier for sperm. The best way to consume grapefruit juice, of course, is to make your own and there are some great low cost juicers on the market.

Sperm cells love environments that are alkaline (high pH). The pH of your cervical mucous is caused by the overall pH level in your body, most of which is the result of your diet. Eating a healthy diet that's high in dark green vegetables, lima beans, almonds, citrus fruits, and other alkaline goods will help make your cervical mucous more sperm-friendly. Try to limit any foods that are processed such as refined grains, most meat, and sugar since these are acidifying.

Achieve a healthy weight

A healthy weight is important if you're trying to conceive. If you're even a few pounds underweight or overweight, it can affect your ability to conceive. The ideal BMI for conception is 20 to 25. Being either underweight or overweight can cause problems with ovulation.

Excess body fat can cause an overproduction of certain hormones that can disturb ovulation. This can lead to irregular cycles and cycles in which you aren't ovulating at all. If you are overweight, even losing just 5% of your body weight can boost chances of conceiving by about a fifth.

You don't want to be underweight either, if you can help it. If you have too little body fat then your body may not produce the hormones it needs to ovulate every month. If your doctor believes you are underweight then gaining as few as 5 pounds might be enough to help trigger your cycles to becoming more regular.

Diet

It is important to eat a healthy diet, even before you start trying to conceive again, but especially while you are pregnant.

A lot of doctors think a healthy diet can boost fertility, especially if you are suffering from certain ovulation issues such as ovulatory dysfunction or sub clinical PCOS (polycystic ovary syndrome).

Tips for a healthy diet include:

Protein. It is important to include protein in a healthy diet, though a lot of Westerners eat too much and rely too much on chicken, beef, and pork for it. The amount of protein on your plate should be about the size of a pack of playing cards. The authorities at Harvard Medical School recommend replacing a serving of meat every day with protein such as tofu, beans, peas, or nuts as this can boost fertility.

Fresh fruits. Most fresh fruits are considered very healthy though try not to eat too much as they do still contain sugar. Those that contain vitamin B6, like bananas, can help regulate hormones. A B6 deficiency has been linked to poor sperm quality and irregular cycles. Berries are particularly good for fertility as they contain anti-oxidants which may help with egg quality and strawberries also contain folic acid.

Hydration. It is important to stay hydrated and drink plenty of water. Water helps create a strong supply of blood to the uterus' lining. In addition, staying hydrated will ensure that your cervical mucus, which helps the sperm to the egg, is fast moving.

Fiber. Fiber can help regulate blood sugar levels, which can reduce fertility issues and promote healthy hormonal balance. High fiber foods include dark leafy greens, fruits, vegetables, beans, and whole grains - bread where you can actually see the bits of grains in there.

Calcium. Include milk, cheese and yogurt in your diet but eat organic versions wherever possible. A Harvard University study discovered that women who eat at least one serving of full-fat dairy every day can reduce their risk of infertility by more than 25%. Dairy can also encourage the ovaries to work more efficiently.

Iron. Iron is important in your overall health but a deficiency can also specifically impact fertility. Women who suffer from anemia may have lack of ovulation and poor egg health. This can hinder pregnancy at a rate that is 60% higher than those who are not anemic. Sources of iron include navy beans, tofu, lentils, kidney beans, molasses, spinach, and raw pumpkin seeds.

Colorful vegetables. Colorful vegetables offer a lot of vitamins and minerals and contain phytochemicals and antioxidants, which destroy free radicals and toxins. Free radicals can cause harm to the reproductive system, including sperm count. Some of the best vegetables are the ones that are brightly colored, such as red peppers and spinach. It is suggested that you try to eat at least 7 portions of brightly colored vegetables a day for optimum fertility. This might sound a lot but if you have a salad you can include 4 or 5 in one go.

Alkaline foods. Alkaline foods can determine your internal pH balance, which can affect your fertility. Most American diets are acid-forming since they contain a lot of meats, sugar, white flour, pastas, trans-fats, and dairy. Those who have highly stressful lives also tend to have acidity, too, since stress can affect the pH balance.

In an acidic environment, micro-organisms like yeast and other unhealthy bacteria can thrive. Some of these hinder the absorption of the essential vitamins and minerals that are in charge of the hormonal balance responsible for healthy reproduction and fertility. A very acidic environment can cause many fertility concerns such as vaginal infections, menstrual irregularities, urinary tract infections, prostatitis, infertility, and impotence.

Sperm prefer an alkaline environment and an alkaline diet can improve the quality of cervical mucus making it more sperm friendly. Foods to consume include papaya, spinach, kale, other leafy green vegetables, avocado, red peppers, wheatgrass, lemon-infused water, nuts, peas, sweet potatoes and olive oil. These will help create a more alkaline environment, which can naturally boost fertility.

It is also possible to invest in water cartridges or a water filter jug, which will help make your tap water alkaline. Biocera is a good company to investigate if you are interested in this http://www.biocera.com.

Avoid acidic foods. Acidic foods, such as most processed foods, alcohol, and coffee can make your cervical mucus hostile to sperm.

Do a body detox

Sometimes, a simply body detox or fertility cleanse can be enough to jump-start your system and get everything in the reproductive system in working order. With all the chemicals in our food and toxins in the environment these days, there's quite a bit of toxicity in the body. This can decrease the quality of sperm and eggs and cause hormonal problems in both men and women. If you had methotrexate treatment then a detox can be especially helpful to clear the drugs from your system before you try to conceive again.

A detox doesn't have to be complicated and doesn't have to take long. Some people do a detox for 24 hours while others do them for a three or five day period. There are also "lifestyle" detoxes, which carry on for a month or more and consist of removing or eliminating certain foods, ingredients, or products from the diet in order to live a healthier lifestyle.

Some detoxes are more extreme than others and involve just juices and light vegetable broths for a period of time, others just recommend following a set of guidelines to give your body a rest from the most taxing things we digest. It's always a good idea to talk to a medical practitioner if you want to undertake a more extreme detox.

We've included some to-do's for a mild detox below:

Sample Dietary Cleanse

Length: 3-10 Days

Goal: To increase bile production to make the liver more efficient and remove toxins from the body.

Foods to Avoid

Alcohol – It probably goes without saying but studies have shown that even light alcohol consumption can have a negative effect on fertility and fertility treatments. You should definitely cut it out during a detox and if you do drink consider giving up completely (or almost completely) whilst trying to conceive.

Caffeine – Caffeine is popular, but it's not healthy. It can cause headaches, fatigue, and withdrawal symptoms when you give it up. It can also give us irregular energy and push us when our bodies really need to be resting, not to mention the damage it can do to our teeth enamel.

Sugar – Refined sugar is difficult for our bodies to digest and it depletes the body of nutrients. Many nutritionists are now starting to claim that sugar should be drastically reduced in our diets permanently and it is certainly one to restrict for optimum fertility.

Gluten – Gluten can be difficult for people to digest. It contains enzyme inhibitors that can cause difficulties such as bloating, constipation, diarrhea, and even rashes and fatigue.

Meat – Although meat is full of protein and is nutrient dense, from time to time it's important to take a break from it. Red meat, especially, can be extremely high in cholesterol and difficult for our bodies to digest. Finding other forms of protein to give our bodies energy is preferable during this time period.

Dairy – In general women who have one portion of full-fat dairy a day benefit from increased fertility but during a detox it's good to give your body a rest as processing dairy is harder for our bodies than other foods.

Foods to Include

Probiotics - Probiotic supplements give your body the good bacteria it needs for a healthy digestive system. Including a good probiotic supplement will keep your immune system up and running and to cut down on bloating, nausea, and constipation.

Vegetables – These should form your main food group during a detox. Eat a wide range of colors with a mix of lightly steamed and raw. Juicing vegetables also helps your body digest them and if you're considering a detox and more healthy living generally then investing in a juicer is worthwhile. It's also fine to drink fruit juice whilst detoxing but try to keep the majority of the juice vegetable, perhaps adding an apple to keep the juice sweet.

Homemade broth - Cooking at home is almost always healthier than eating out, but homemade broths made from vegetable stocks or even chicken bones contain a lot of minerals and can help enrich the digestive system.

Seafood - Wild seafood, not farmed, has a lot of healthy nutrients. Wild salmon, especially, is rich with amino acids, which can help protect against everything from heart attacks to strokes and has been known to be great for the complexion. Some people prefer to be completely vegetarian or even vegan during their detoxes but if that is too much for you to bear then a small amount of fish is ok.

Berries - Berries are nature's natural sweeteners. They are low in sugar and can naturally cleanse the body. Some berries (blueberries, strawberries, and raspberries) also contain a lot of antioxidants, which can fight damage caused by free radicals.

Other detox tips

It is recommended that you seek professional help before starting a detox and that you don't go into or come out of a detox too quickly as your body won't be able to handle that well. There are some other things to bear in mind with a detox:

- o It may be obvious but even with the things you've decided you will still eat – vegetables and perhaps some fish for example – make sure you don't eat too much. The idea is to give your body a break.

- o Don't let your blood sugar drop too long so ensure you have regular snacks - such as nuts or carrot sticks or a juice every three hours or so.

- o Don't eat late – try to have your last meal or juice of the day before 6.30pm which again will take the pressure off your digestive system.

- o If the detox is going to be hard for you then perhaps persuade your partner to do it with you – it can only help his fertility too.

- o Be kind to yourself – many people experience headaches from the withdrawal of both caffeine and sugar but if you can last these should disappear within a few days and your body will really thank you for the break. You may find it much easier to restrict or even remove these from your diet post detox.

- o You'll probably be more tired than normal so plan your detox for when you don't have much other activity on and go to bed early.

- o Some people find themselves getting tearful or emotional during a detox – don't worry if this happens to you – it's just part of the process.

- o Do partake of some light exercise – gentle yoga or walks in nature can really help the process and keep your mood positive.

A detox can be a great investment in your health generally, even if you just decide to cut out some of the more toxic elements of your diet for a week or so, your fertility should experience a boost.

Boost progesterone levels

Although your doctor can give you supplements for progesterone if your levels are low, there are also some natural methods of your boosting your levels as well. These include:

- Increasing the intake of foods that are rich in vitamin B.

- Eating a diet low in meats and animal by-products, since a lot of times the hormones given to them can act as estrogens in your body.

- Forgoing plastics, canned foods, or conventional cleaners and beauty products whenever possible. A lot of them contain estrogen-like compounds that cause a body to become estrogen dominant.

- Make sure you're getting enough magnesium – if you are deficient this can have a big impact on fertility. A magnesium supplement (ideally 400mg per day) can help boost fertility and also prevent SIDS when your baby is born.

- Get adequate amounts of protein every day from either organic or grass fed meat sources or vegetable sources. For production, hormones need adequate protein.

- Eat a lot of vegetables, especially leafy green and bright orange ones. The micro-nutrients they contain are essential for progesterone production. Some studies show that both sweet potatoes and yams can help the body produce progesterone and even reduce the risk of miscarriage when you do become pregnant.

- If you use a progesterone cream, use one that is bio-identical like one from Beeyoutiful.

- Make sure you're not experiencing adrenal fatigue. Have your cortisol levels checked. When your adrenal glands are fatigued the antecedent to progesterone is used to make cortisol instead of progesterone. An adrenal saliva test can show you what your cortisol levels are. Supplements can help you fight adrenal fatigue.

Limit exposure to chemicals

Try to avoid or limit the following ingredients in your body care products because they can lower your fertility by disrupting your hormones, including progesterone and estrogen:

- Dibutyl Phthalate

- Sodium Lauryl Sulphate in your shampoo

- Mineral Oil in creams

- Petroleum in many personal care products

- Sodium Fluoride in your toothpaste

- Diethanolamine and triethanolamine

- Propylene glycol

- Parabens in most shampoos, conditioner and creams

- Diazolidinyl Urea

- Benzoic Acid

- Isopropyl Alcohol

- Any fragrances

If time allows you might consider learning to make your own cleaning supplies and beauty products. It's not as hard as it sounds. For instance, a fast and fun body scrub can be made by adding brown sugar, olive oil, lavender essential oil, and vitamin E oil in a container. Plus, it costs a fraction of the amount you would have paid in a store.

When you're buying your personal care products, look for those that are organic and ideally paraben-free. Parabens are a common toxin that can be found in many different personal care products, such as shampoos and lotions as mentioned above. Parabens are a preservative and keep products from spoiling. However, when the body absorbs them, they can imitate estrogen. As a result, there is some concern that they might be dangerous to the reproductive system and hamper fertility.

Two companies that make good products that fit these guidelines are:

Jason

http://www.jason-personalcare.com

and

Green People (they deliver worldwide)
http://www.greenpeople.co.uk

And there are other similar companies to be found online with just a little investigation.

Learn to relax

Too much stress can be detrimental to the body if you're trying to conceive. Stress affects both partners' fertility by causing a disruption in the hormonal balance. During stress, the body feels the pressure physically and emotionally. This may cause internal organs to work harder than normal and can even affect hormonal output. For some women, their menstrual cycle might be affected and they could find that their egg release is inhibited. In extremely stressful situations, testosterone levels and reduced sperm production has been seen in men. A study published in the June 2011 publication of Fertility and Sterility found that women who took part in a mind/body therapy program while undergoing IVF faired considerably better than those who didn't participate. Fifty-two percent of the women in the program conceived, compared to only 20% of the women who didn't participate.

Of course if you're trying to conceive following an ectopic pregnancy that in itself can be incredibly stressful. You may even find you start to live your life with mood swings that accompany your monthly cycle – going from hope and excitement in the first half of your cycle to worry and nerves during the last week as you wait (or don't wait!) to test and then utter disappointment when and if your bleeding begins each month. It might be helpful to realize that many, many women experience the same thing and whilst it is utterly exhausting whilst you're in this phase you will forget this stressful part of your life when you finally hold your baby in your arms.

When you're trying to conceive, everyone tells you not to become stressed and this can be incredibly frustrating as fertility issues are one of the most stressful experiences you may go through. Try to stay sane when you're given this advice – unless someone has been through the process of trying to conceive for a long time, they're unlikely to appreciate the impact their comments are having!

Having said all this - learning some stress relieving techniques can really help you cope. The following is a list of some activities that might be useful in helping you relax and thus helping you conceive.

Acupuncture

Acupuncture is a Traditional Chinese Medicine (TCM) technique that involves placing very thin needles into specific acupressure points in the body to lessen stress and treat various mental and physical conditions such as chronic pain, depression, nausea and even boost fertility. According to TCM, the body has different channels of energy (called meridians) that flow throughout the body. If one of these becomes blocked or imbalanced there can be a negative effect on your health.

By inserting the needles along the different acupressure points, the nervous system can be stimulated and the flow of energy through that meridian can be improved. Some studies on acupuncture have shown that it can improve blood flow to the uterus and ovaries, and this may stimulate ovulation and even help with implantation.

In one study published in April 2002 in *Fertility and Sterility*, a group of German researchers studied 160 women and discovered that adding acupuncture to the traditional IVF treatment protocols considerably increased pregnancy success. One group of 80 women received two, 25-minute acupuncture treatments. The second group of 80 women, who also underwent embryo transfer, did not receive any acupuncture treatments. Although women in both groups conceived, the rate was considerably higher in those who received acupuncture - 34 pregnancies, compared to the 21 pregnancies in the women who only received IVF. Other studies have shown comparable results.

Massage

A simple good massage can really help you relax. A study published in a 2004 issue of the *International Journal of*

Neurosciences, found that massage also greatly reduce stress. You don't have to have a long massage in order to experience the benefits of it, either. In just a 10 minute treatment, the subjects in this particular study experienced a decrease in anxiety.

A gentle stomach massage during ovulation might help boost fertility by helping position the uterus in the optimal position and remove blockages that might exist in the fallopian tubes. In an article entitled "Gynecologists Investigate Massage As Infertility Treatment" on Personal MD, early research showed a remarkable reversal in 75% of infertility cases that showed tubal blockages (Gynecologists Investigate Massage as Infertility Treatment, 2000). There are specialists who can carry out this type of massage or you can learn how to massage your tummy for increased fertility yourself one from various online sites including Youtube.

https://www.youtube.com/watch?v=UpJLfLHe0B0

This is something that you might want to experiment with along with your partner. Invest in some massage therapy books and practice on one another for some mutual stress relief!

A few benefits of a fertility massage can include:

•   Improved digestion

•   Increased blood flow to the reproductive organs

•   Reduced inflammation that can be caused by ovarian cysts or uterine fibroids

Yoga

Yoga is known for being an invigorating exercise, increasing mindfulness and a relaxing activity all in one. It can also boost fertility by offering you poses that can help support and strengthen the endocrine and reproductive systems. The endocrine system is important for good hormonal balance. Yoga can also increase circulation to your reproductive system, support a healthy immune system, and possibly help remove blockages that are present in the reproductive areas.

It's hard to deny the benefits that come with the relaxation that yoga offers. Many people enjoy it simply for the fact that it provides mediation and centering activity that helps them de-stress.

If yoga is new to you then you might want to go with a beginner's class, or a gentle style such as Kripalu or basic Hatha. Other styles such as Ashtanga or Bikram can be more energetic and are usually more suited for those who are more advanced or in pretty good physical shape to begin with.

Yoga classes can be found at a community center, local college or university, gym, YMCA, or fitness center. Some fitness centers allow you to pay by the class so that you don't have to buy an entire membership to the center. This might also work out to be a little more budget-friendly.

Drink more herbal tea

Certain teas are not only tasty, but can help boost your fertility as well. The following are a couple of teas that are known for their reproductive perks.

Green tea

Green tea might be a caffeinated drink, but unlike other caffeinated beverages, it's actually good for you in small quantities. It contains a lot of different types of antioxidants and these may give your immune system a boost. Although scientists aren't sure why green tea helps when it comes to conceiving, the protective properties in green tea can't hurt and the Chinese have been using it in Traditional Chinese Medicine (TCM) for hundreds of years for fertility issues.

One study carried out by the Kaiser Permanent Medical Care Program discovered that women who drank green tea regularly doubled their chances of conceiving. Keep in mind, however, that too much green tea may interfere with folic acid absorption. It's also important to limit the consumption of green tea to two cups per day since any more caffeine than that has been linked to increased miscarriage rates.

Red raspberry leaf

Red raspberry leaf has been used in Native American cultures for many years as a natural fertility treatment as a way to strengthen the lining of the uterus. Today, we know that this may help with implantation. Red raspberry leaf might also lengthen the luteal phase and improve blood circulation in the reproductive organs.

Normally, this leaf is brewed into a tea. It can be sweetened with honey and consumed throughout the cycle. There's no limit to how many glasses you can drink a day. Some women even drink it at the end of their pregnancy to help prepare their uterus for contractions since it can help strengthen the muscles and "tone" the uterus. However, once you get a positive pregnancy test, you shouldn't drink red raspberry leaf tea until the third trimester because it does have uterine toning effects and until the end of the third trimester your uterus needs to remain soft and supple so that it can stretch and grow along with your baby.

Drink Lemon water

Lemons are tart and sour but they're good for you. They contain a lot of vitamin C and antioxidants that help flush out your system and improve your overall health. Lemons are an alkalinizing food. Since your vaginal environment is naturally acidic and hostile to sperm, lemons can make your vagina more alkaline and more accepting to the sperm. You can add lemons to your diet by squeezing half a lemon into a cup of warm water and drinking this about 15 minutes in the morning before you eat anything. If you're not keen on the lemon water, you can also try squeezing it into green tea.

Herbs

Before modern medicine developed the drugs we have today, practitioners treated most of our ailments with herbal remedies and this practice is still used effectively in many parts of the world. This includes infertility. If you decide to use any natural supplements then you should talk to a health practitioner first, especially if you're already taking any other medication or are undergoing any fertility treatments since even natural supplements can interact with these. Most of the time, it is not recommended that women take fertility drugs and herbal supplements simultaneously.

Remember, too, that although herbs are natural substances, they are still very powerful medicines and as such can have serious side effects. Your medical practitioner can ensure that you take the correct herbs to assist you and discuss the quantities that match your needs. If you start having any side effects, you can then discuss these with a professional and see if any changes need to be made.

Some of the herbs recommended for boosting fertility are:

Black Cohosh: an antispasmodic (keeps the muscles from spasming) herb that can relieve menstrual cramps and may stimulate the ovaries. You should only take it only during the first half of your menstrual cycle and stop taking it after ovulation.

Evening Primrose Oil: EPO has been known to improve the quality of cervical mucus by making it thinner and more watery. It should also be stopped after ovulation since it can cause uterine contractions, which could endanger an implanted embryo.

Chaste Berry (Vitex): also known as the "female herb," this herb can help regulate hormones. Scientists think it affects the pituitary gland and hypothalamus, which regulate the hormones involved in reproduction. It may strengthen ovulation by causing an increase in LH production. It's safe to use it at any time during your cycle but you should stop it once you have a positive pregnancy test. It also shouldn't be taken continuously for longer than six months since it can reduce your body's prolactin levels and when these are too high, menstruation can become irregular.

False Unicorn: a root, False Unicorn is meant to be used before ovulation begins and during the luteal phase. It is meant to help regulate the ovaries. It should not be taken throughout the pregnancy so it must be stopped once you've had a positive pregnancy test.

Turmeric: a herb often found in curry, Turmeric is known to naturally help increase the body's progesterone levels which can help boost fertility and maintain pregnancies.

Maca: Maca is known around the world for its fertility and vitality promoting properties. It should only be taken between menstruation and ovulation and not taken during pregnancy. Maca can also be hugely beneficial for improving your partner's fertility too.

It can be overwhelming to find the herbs that work best for you or even knowing where to start. Finding a registered medical herbalist, or a naturopath, who will talk to you and take a comprehensive medical history will help you make the right herbal choices based on your health and fertility issues. When you're talking to him or her, it's important to tell them about any other medications you're taking. This way, you'll hopefully avoid any harmful interactions.

Unlike a lot of medications that are out today, most herbs do not work instantaneously. Herbs have a cumulative effect and it may take them weeks or a couple of months to work with your body's chemistry and have an impact on your fertility. Also remember to ask which herbs you are taking should be stopped once you become pregnant since they might be harmful to a developing baby.

Soy isoflavones

Clomid is one of the most popular fertility treatments available. Many women opt not to undergo this treatment, however, due to the risks associated with it. It does have a possible risk of ectopic pregnancy, too, and if you've already suffered from an ectopic pregnancy this is something you might want to keep under consideration. Soy isoflavones can produce a similar reaction to Clomid and are seen by many as a natural alternative.

Clomid isn't an estrogen but has a similar structure; it binds to the estrogen receptor cells in the hypothalamus (the part of the brain responsible for hormone production) and blocks them. When your estrogen receptor cells are blocked, the brain doesn't get the signal from the estrogen. Although your estrogen levels aren't low, your body thinks they are. This is important since estrogen is released from your follicles as they mature. If your follicles don't mature then you aren't able to ovulate. Clomid blocks your estrogen receptors and confuses your body into thinking you need more *Follicle Stimulating Hormone* (FSH).

The *Gonadotropin-releasing hormone* (GNRH) stimulates the production of FSH. When the estrogen levels are low, GNRH production increases. GNRH stimulates the FSH and the FSH stimulates your follicles. As your follicles mature they release the estrogen. When your estrogen reaches a certain level, your body will ovulate. Because FSH is the hormone that makes your follicles mature, Clomid can confuse your body into producing more FSH and so it will hopefully either stimulate or improve ovulation.

Soy isoflavones are known as "phytoestrogens" called Selective Estrogen Receptor Modulators (SERM). Clomid is a SERM, too. Many people think that because soy isoflavones are also a SERM, they can function in the same way as Clomid. Soy isoflavones have been found to bind to estrogen receptors, although the bind is weak. Still, it's possible that soy isoflavones can work as a natural ovulation stimulator. However, more studies are needed in this area.

For soy isoflavones to work in a manner that is similar to Clomid's strength, they should be taken for about five days at the start of a cycle. They would usually be taken either on days 3-7 or 5-9, the same as one would take Clomid. Most of the women who take soy isoflavones to stimulate ovulation take around 150-200 mg a day on these days. However, keep in mind that since there haven't been any scientific studies on the effects of soy isoflavones and ovulation, these guidelines are just general and based on Clomid's recommendations. The dosage should not be continued throughout the cycle because it can hinder ovulation.

If you have problems with your thyroid, you should probably avoid soy isoflavones since soy products can aggravate thyroid conditions. Some evidence also suggests that high levels of soy consumption might decrease fertility. While some soy isoflavones may work as an estrogen blocker, others may mimic estrogen. As of now, there aren't enough published studies out there to say how taking isoflavones daily can affect fertility. If you're interested in soy isoflavones it's probably a good idea to do some more research and to find a health specialist who can help you.

Limit Caffeine

When you're trying to conceive, you should try to stay away from or limit your caffeine intake as much as possible. More than 2 cups of caffeine per day has been linked to a higher risk of miscarriage. However, studies have been inconclusive as far as whether or not caffeine can actually affect infertility (Anderson et al 2010, NCCWCH 2013: 70), although a few small studies have found that women who consumed more than 2 cups of coffee per day have more trouble getting pregnant than women who don't drink caffeine.

If you're having IVF treatments, then caffeine definitely needs to be limited. Caffeine ingestion of more than 2mg to 50mg per day on a regular basis has been linked to a lower success rate for IVF (NCCWCH 2013:228).

More research needs to be done but limiting caffeine does have health and fertility benefits.

Conclusion

There's no doubt that an ectopic pregnancy is a devastating diagnosis. Whilst it's true that women are no longer in mortal danger from an ectopic pregnancy, when you've been through something so traumatic, especially if it was a longed for child, then this may seem like cold comfort.

It's imperative that you and your partner allow yourselves to grieve for your loss and that you give your body, and of course emotions, some time to recover. There are most definitely things you can do to help your recovery and hopefully this book will help you form an idea of what could work best for you. Whilst some women find it useful to have a plan mapped out to help them, others prefer to go with the flow. What's important is that you do what feels right for you and that you use this time to go easy on yourself. Sometimes a bottle of wine and a takeaway are exactly what's needed and you certainly shouldn't feel bad about doing what's comforting to you.

If you do want to try to conceive again the waiting time can feel incredibly long and frustrating but there is so much you can do to use this time positively. Doctors are only now beginning to understand and appreciate just how much a woman's diet in the months leading up to conception, for example, can impact on a baby's health for life.

If and when you feel up to it, use the down time to do as much as you can to get your body in to the best shape for pregnancy – eating good food mindfully, taking some exercise and actively looking for ways to reduce the stress in your life. You can use this time to create healthy habits that will stand you in good stead not just for the rest of your life, but for the rest of your future children's lives too.

Remember that whilst the emotional pain of an ectopic pregnancy may always remain with you that you are not alone. Recovering is not instantaneous but it will happen and it is within your gift to replace your own natural fear and uncertainty with knowledge and positive action.

Helpful Websites

Ectopic Pregnancy

The Ectopic Pregnancy Trust

http://www.ectopic.org.uk/patients/

Mayo Clinic's Ectopic Pregnancy Page

http://www.mayoclinic.org/diseases-conditions/ectopic-pregnancy/basics/definition/con-20024262

March of Dimes: Ectopic and molar pregnancy

http://www.marchofdimes.com/loss/ectopic-and-molar-pregnancy.aspx

American Pregnancy Association: Ectopic Pregnancy

http://americanpregnancy.org/pregnancycomplications/ectopicpregnancy.html

Ectopic Pregnancy Foundation

http://www.ectopicpregnancyfoundation.org/

Ectopic Pregnancy: NHS Choices

http://www.nhs.uk/conditions/ectopic-pregnancy/Pages/Introduction.aspx

Ectopic pregnancy information

http://www.patient.co.uk/health/ectopic-pregnancy-leaflet

The American Society for Reproductive Medicine

http://www.asrm.org/Ectopic_Pregnancy_factsheet/

Ectopic Pregnancy: Tommy's

http://www.tommys.org/ectopic

Endometriosis

Endometriosis.org

http://endometriosis.org/support/support-groups/

Endometriosis Research Center

https://www.endocenter.org/

WebMD Support Group

http://exchanges.webmd.com/endometriosis

Endometriosis UK

http://www.endometriosis-uk.org/

The Endometriosis Association

http://www.endometriosisassn.org/

Online Support Groups

Ectopic Pregnancy: Baby Center: New Hopes:
http://community.babycenter.com/groups/a734235/ectopic
pregnancy-_new_hopes

Ectopic Pregnancy & Miscarriage Support: Café Mom:
http://www.cafemom.com/group/23916

Ectopic Pregnancy Trust: http://www.ectopic.org.uk/talk/

BabyCenter's Ectopic & Molar Board (US):
http://community.babycenter.com/groups/a113685/molar_
and_partial_molar_pregnancies

BabyCenter's Ectopic & Molar Board (UK):
http://community.babycentre.co.uk/groups/a62945/ectopic
_molar_board

Hyster Sisters

An active online forum and information site relating to hysterectomies.

www.hystersisters.com

Silent Grief - online chat board for those who have lost pregnancies and infants

http://www.silentgrief.com/

Charities

Hannah's Prayer Ministries- offering support for fertility challenges - http://www.hannah.org/

Hygeia Foundation- supporting the loss of a pregnancy or infant - http://hygeiafoundation.org/

March of Dimes - Ectopic and Molar Pregnancy page- http://www.marchofdimes.com/loss/ectopic-and-molar-pregnancy.aspx

The Ectopic Pregnancy Foundation

http://www.ectopicpregnancy.co.uk/

Ectopic Pregnancy Ireland

http://ectopicireland.ie/

Relaxation Specialists

Acupuncture

The Acupuncture Society

www.acupuncturesociety.org.uk

The British Medical Acupuncture Society

www.medical-acupuncture.co.uk/

The British Acupuncture Council

www.acupuncture.org.uk/

Acupuncture Society of America, Inc

www.acupuncturesociety.org/

Acupuncture-Gateway to Chinese Medicine, Health, & Wellness

http://www.acupuncture.com/

Massage therapy

National Certified Board for Therapeutic Massage and Body Work-find a therapist (US)

http://www.ncbtmb.org/tools/find-a-certified-massage-therapist

Alternative Medicines: Natural Therapy Pages (UK)

http://www.naturaltherapypages.co.uk/

Complementary Therapy Resource (UK)

http://massagetherapy.co.uk/directory/

Where to Buy…

Ovulation Kits

Fertile Focus: http://www.fairhavenhealth.com/fertile-focus.html

First Response Easy Read Ovulation Test: http://www.firstresponse.com/ovulation-test.asp

Clearblue Easy Digital Ovulation Test UK: http://uk.clearblue.com/clearblue-ovulation-test-range/clearblue-digital-ovulation-test-%E2%80%93-7-test-pack

True Ultra Sensitive Ovulation Test Strips (30 pack) UK:
http://www.amazon.co.uk/True-Sensitive-Ovulation-Fertility-Approved/dp/B00GFP4ZG4

Natural Progesterone Cream

Natural Progesterone Cream

Beeyootiful Balance:
http://www.beeyoutiful.com/beeyoutiful-balance.html

Nature's Sunshine:
http://www.naturessunshine.com/us/general/search/?q=progesterone+cream

Progesterone All Natural Balancing Cream:
http://www.progesterall.com/index.html

Glossary of Terms

Abdominal pregnancy. An ectopic pregnancy that has implanted in an organ or tissue in the abdomen rather than the ovaries, uterus, or fallopian tubes.

Adenomyosis. The uterine thickening that occurs when endometrial tissue, which usually lines the uterus, moves into the outer muscular walls (myometrium) of the uterus.

Adhesiolysis. The removal or surgical separation of adhesions.

Anovulation. A cycle during which the ovaries do not release an egg, thus meaning that complete ovulation doesn't take place.

Appendicitis. A medical condition in which the appendix (a tubular organ attached to the colon) becomes infected and inflamed. It can be associated with the formation of adhesions in the immediacy of the fallopian tubes.

Cervix. The lower part of the uterus that connects the uterus to the vagina.

Corpus luteum. The discarded tissue that is left behind after the egg is released from the ovary. It secretes progesterone. If an egg isn't fertilized, the corpus luteum stays for about 13 or 14 days and maintains progesterone levels that keep the uterine lining thick. After that it disintegrates and progesterone levels gradually drop until the uterine lining can't be sustained. The lining is then shed, and the woman has menstruation. If the egg is fertilized, the corpus luteum provides the signal so that when the fertilized egg reaches the uterus, the lining is prepared to accept it and implantation can occur. If pregnancy occurs, the progesterone that is secreted by the corpus luteum maintains the uterine lining for 8-10 weeks. After that, the placenta takes over the production.

Diethylstilbestrol (DES). A synthetic hormone that was once given to women during early pregnancy to prevent miscarriage. Its use was stopped in the 1970s since studies discovered that women born from treated pregnancies can have abnormalities of the reproductive system, amongst other problems.

Dilation and curettage (D&C). A surgical procedure in which the cervix is dilated and the lining of the uterus is scraped away. Afterwards, the tissue is examined for the presence of abnormalities.

Ectopic pregnancy. A pregnancy that implants outside of the uterus, usually in one of the fallopian tubes. Also referred to as a "tubal pregnancy" since the majority of ectopic pregnancies occur within the fallopian tubes. Ectopic means "out of place."

Embryo. The earliest stage of human development; generally the name given to a developing fetus immediately after the fertilization of the sperm and the egg takes place.

Endometriosis. A condition in which patches of endometrial-like tissue develop outside the uterine cavity in irregular locations such as the ovaries, bowels, fallopian tubes, and abdominal cavity. Endometriosis can grow and cause pain and inflammation and lead to infertility. It is a risk factor associated with ectopic pregnancy.

Endometrium. The inner mucous membrane of the uterus.

Fallopian tube. A pair of hollow tubes that are attached one on each side of the uterus. The egg travels from the ovary to the uterus through the fallopian tubes and fertilization normally occurs here. The fallopian tube is the most frequent site of ectopic pregnancies.

Fertility drugs. Medications that stimulate the ovaries to produce and mature eggs so that they will be released during ovulation.

Fimbriae. The finger-like fringed ends of the fallopian tubes that sweep over the ovary and help guide the egg into the tube.

Heterotopic pregnancy. When both a viable embryo exists within the uterus and an ectopic pregnancy is implanted outside of the uterus at the same time.

Human chorionic gonadotropin (hCG). The hormone produced by the placenta during pregnancy.

Implantation. The process in which an embryo pushes itself into the uterine lining to gain nourishment and oxygen. In an ectopic pregnancy, an embryo will implant somewhere outside of the uterus, such as in the fallopian tube or on the ovary.

In vitro fertilization (IVF). A fertility procedure that involves combining an egg with sperm in a laboratory dish. If fertilization occurs and cell division begins then the embryo is transferred into the uterus where it will implant in the uterine lining. In some cases, IVF is performed along with medications that stimulate the ovaries to produce multiple eggs to boost the chances of fertilization and implantation. The incentive of IVF is that it circumvents the fallopian tubes which can be ideal for those who are missing tubes or have tubes that are damaged.

Laparoscope. A thin, lighted, instrument that is usually inserted through the belly button into the stomach to inspect the pelvic and abdominal cavities. The laparoscope is used as both a diagnostic and operative tool.

Laparoscopy. A surgery in which a laparoscope is inserted through a small incision, generally through the belly button, and additional small incisions are also made in the abdominal cavity to allow the entrance of other small instruments. This allows diagnosis and surgical correction of abnormalities. The surgeon is able to remove scar tissue and open closed fallopian tubes during this procedure, as well as remove ectopic pregnancies and perform other surgeries with a shorter recovery time than traditional abdominal surgery.

Laparotomy. A major abdominal surgery in which an incision is made in the abdominal wall. Recovery time is longer than with a laparoscopy.

Luteal phase. The part of the menstrual cycle that begins at ovulation and stops the first day of the woman's period.

Methotrexate. A medication often used to treat ectopic pregnancies since it can eliminate pregnancy-related tissue and quicken the re-absorption of this tissue.

Microsurgery. Surgery that uses magnification, careful technique, and fine suture material in order to get precise surgical results. This kind of surgery is especially important for certain types of tubal surgery in women, particularly when repairing fallopian tubes after the removal of an ectopic pregnancy.

Miscarriage. The naturally occurring discharge of a nonviable fetus and placenta from the uterus. Miscarriage can also be medically known as a "spontaneous abortion" or pregnancy loss.

Myomectomy: A myomectomy is often used to remove fibroids from the uterus. Adhesions can form along the incision line on the uterus as a complication.

Ovaries. The two female sex glands in the pelvis, located one on either side of the uterus. Ovaries are responsible for producing the eggs and hormones including estrogen, progesterone, and androgen.

Partial salpingectomy. A surgery in which the section of a fallopian tube that contains an ectopic pregnancy is removed. This surgery is an attempt to maintain as much of the tube as possible for subsequent re-attachment using microsurgery for women who wish to conceive in the future.

Progesterone. A female hormone that is secreted by the corpus luteum after ovulation during the second half of the menstrual cycle. Progesterone prepares the lining of the uterus for the implantation of a fertilized egg. It also allows for complete shedding of the endometrium during menstruation.

Salpingectomy. A surgery in which one or both of the fallopian tubes are removed.

Salpingitis. An infection and inflammation in the fallopian tubes.

Salpingo-oophorectomy. A surgery in which both the fallopian tube and ovary are removed.

Salpingotomy. A surgery in which the wall of the fallopian tube is opened and the ectopic pregnancy is removed. The incision is left to heal on its own.

Sexually transmitted disease (STD). An infection, such as chlamydia or gonorrhea, that is transmitted by sexual activity. Some STDs in women can cause pelvic infections and lead to infertility by damaging and scarring the fallopian tubes and increasing the risk of ectopic pregnancy.

Transvaginal ultrasound. A test that is used to look at a woman's reproductive organs, including the uterus, ovaries, and cervix. A small probe is inserted into the vagina and the pelvic region is displayed on a video screen.

Tubal ligation. A surgery in which the fallopian tubes are clamped, clipped, or cut in order to prevent pregnancy.

Ultrasound. An image of internal organs that is produced by high frequency sound waves viewed as an image on a video screen. Ultrasounds are used to monitor growth of ovarian follicles, retrieve eggs, or monitor the growth and development of a fetus.

Uterus (womb). The hollow, muscular female organ in the pelvis where an embryo implants and grows. The lining of the uterus is called the endometrium and it produces the monthly menstrual blood flow when pregnancy isn't present.

Studies

Abbott J, Emmans LS, Lowenstein SR. Ectopic pregnancy: ten common pitfalls in diagnosis. *Am J Emerg Med.* 1990;8:515–22.

Agarwal A, Deepinder F, Cocuzza M, Short RA, Evenson DP. "Effect of vaginal lubricants on sperm motility and chromatin integrity: a prospective comparative study." *Fertility and Sterility.* 2008 Feb;89(2):375-9. Epub 2007 May 16.

Anderson K, Norman RJ, Middleton P. 2010. Preconception lifestyle advice for people with subfertility. Cochrane Database of Systematic Reviews, Issue 4. Art. No.: CD008189. DOI: 10.1002/14651858.CD008189.pub2

Anderson L, Lewis SE, McClure N. "The effects of coital lubricants on sperm motility in vitro." *Human Reproduction.* 1998 Dec;13(12):3351-6.

Barnhart KT, Katz I, Hummel A, & Gracia CR. *Presumed diagnosis of ectopic pregnancy.* Obstet Gynecol. 2002 Sep;100(3):505-10.

D D Baird, C R Weinberg, L F Voigt, and J R Daling. "Vaginal douching and reduced fertility." *American Journal of Public Health.* 1996 June; 86(6): 844-850.

Bak CW, Lyu SW, Seok HH, Byun JS, Lee JH, Shim SH, Yoon TK. "Erectile Dysfunction and Extramarital Sex Induced by Timed Intercourse: A Prospective Study of 439 Men." *Journal of Andrology.* 2012 May 3.

Bangsgaard N, Lund CO, Ottesen B, Nilas L. Improved fertility following conservative surgical treatment of ectopic pregnancy. BJOG 2003; 110:765.

Barnhart KT, Gosman G, Ashby R, Sammel M. The medical management of ectopic pregnancy: a meta-analysis comparing "single dose" and "multidose" regimens. *Obstet Gynecol.* Apr 2003;101(4):778-84.

CDC. Maternal deaths associated with barbiturate anesthetics—New York City. MMWR 1986;35:579–82, 587.

Creanga AA, Shapiro-Mendoza CK, Bish CL, Zane S, Berg CJ, Callaghan WM. Trends in ectopic pregnancy mortality in the United States 1980–2007. Obstet Gynecol 2011;117:837–43.

Dor J, Seidman DS, Levran D, Ben-Rafael Z, Ben-Shlomo I, Mashiach S. The incidence of combined intrauterine and extrauterine pregnancy after in vitro fertilization and embryo transfer. *Fertil Steril.* Apr 1991;55(4):833-4.

Peter M. Doubilet, M.D., Ph.D., Carol B. Benson, M.D., Tom Bourne, M.B., B.S., Ph.D., and Michael Blaivas, M.D. for the Society of Radiologists in Ultrasound Multispecialty Panel on Early First Trimester Diagnosis of Miscarriage and Exclusion of a Viable Intrauterine Pregnancy. *Diagnostic Criteria for Nonviable Pregnancy Early in the First Trimester.* N Engl J Med 2013; 369:1443-1451October 10, 2013 DOI: 10.1056/NEJMra1302417

Dubuisson JB, Morice P, Chapron C, et al. Salpingectomy - the laparoscopic surgical choice for ectopic pregnancy. Hum Reprod 1996; 11:1199.

Ego A, Subtil D, Cosson M, et al. Survival analysis of fertility after ectopic pregnancy. Fertil Steril 2001; 75:560.

Furlong LA. Ectopic pregnancy risk when contraception fails. A review. *J Reprod Med.* Nov 2002;47(11):881-5.

Goldberg, C. (2013, October 11). *Tragically Wrong: When Good Early Pregnancies are Misdiagnosed as Bad.* Retrieved March 4, 2014, from Common Health: http://commonhealth.wbur.org/2013/10/ectopic-pregnancy-misdiagnosed-methotrexate

Gynecologists Investigate Massage as Infertility Treatment . (2000, March 23). Retrieved December 20, 2013, from Personal MD: http://www.personalmd.com/news/n0323123924.shtml

Hajenius PJ, Mol F, Mol BW, et al. Interventions for tubal ectopic pregnancy. Cochrane Database Syst Rev 2007; :CD000324.

Hoover RN, Hyer M, Pfeiffer RM, et al. Adverse health outcomes in women exposed in utero to diethylstilbestrol. *N Engl J Med.* Oct 6 2011;365(14):1304-14.

Hoover KW, Tao G, Kent CK. Trends in the diagnosis and treatment of ectopic pregnancy in the United States. Obstet Gynecol 2010; 115:495–502.

Job-Spira N, Bouyer J, Pouly JL, et al. Fertility after ectopic pregnancy: first results of a population-based cohort study in France. Hum Reprod 1996; 11:99.

Kaplan BC, Dart RG, Moskos M, Kuligowska E, Chun B, Adel Hamid M, et al. Ectopic pregnancy: prospective study with improved diagnostic accuracy. *Ann Emerg Med.* 1996;28:10–7.

Kaunitz AM, Spence C, Danielson TS, Rochat RW, Grimes DA. Perinatal and maternal mortality in a religious group avoiding obstetric care. Am J Obstet Gynecol 1984;150:826–31.

Klonoff-Cohen H. 2005. Female and male lifestyle habits and IVF: what is known and unknown. *Hum. Reprod. Update.* 11(2): 180-204

Kukulu K. "Vaginal douching practices and beliefs in Turkey." *Culture, Health, and Sexuality..* 2006 Jul-Aug;8(4):371-8.

 Kutteh WH, Chao CH, Ritter JO, Byrd W. "Vaginal lubricants for the infertile couple: effect on sperm activity." *International Journal of Fertility and Menopausal Studies.* 1996 Jul-Aug;41(4):400-4.

Lau S, Tulandi T. Conservative medical and surgical management of interstitial ectopic pregnancy. Fertil Steril 1999; 72:207.

Levin, Roy J. "The Physiology of Sexual Arousal in the Human Female: A Recreational and Procreational Synthesis." *Archives of Sexual Behavior.* Volume 31, Number 5, 405-411.

Lundorff P, Thorburn J, Hahlin M, et al. Laparoscopic surgery in ectopic pregnancy. A randomized trial versus laparotomy. Acta Obstet Gynecol Scand 1991; 70:343.

Marion LL, Meeks GR; Ectopic pregnancy: History, incidence, epidemiology, and risk factors. Clin Obstet

Gynecol. 2012 Jun;55(2):376-86. doi: 10.1097/GRF.0b013e3182516d7b.

Michalas S, Minaretzis D, Tsionou C, Maos G, Kioses E, Aravantinos D. First Department of Obstetrics and Gynecology, University of Athens, Alexandra Maternity Hospital, Greece. Pelvic surgery, reproductive factors and risk of ectopic pregnancy: a case controlled study. Int J Gynaecol Obstet. 1992 Jun;38(2):101-5.

Mol BW, Matthijsse HC, Tinga DJ, et al. Fertility after conservative and radical surgery for tubal pregnancy. Hum Reprod 1998; 13:1804.

Murphy AA, Nager CW, Wujek JJ, et al. Operative laparoscopy versus laparotomy for the management of ectopic pregnancy: a prospective trial. Fertil Steril 1992; 57:1180.

NCCWCH. 2013. *Fertility: assessment and treatment for people with fertility problems - full guideline.* National Collaborating Centre for Women's and Children's Health. London: NICE. www.nice.org.uk [pdf file, accessed February 28, 2014]

Paavonen J, et al. (2008). Pelvic inflammatory disease. In KK Holmes et al., eds., Sexually Transmitted Diseases, 4th ed., pp. 1017-1050. New York: McGraw-Hill.

Peterson HB, Xia Z, Hughes JM, Wilcox LS, Tylor LR, Trussell J. The risk of ectopic pregnancy after tubal sterilization. U.S. Collaborative Review of Sterilization Working Group. *N Engl J Med.* Mar 13 1997;336(11):762-7.

Pouly JL, Chapron C, Manhes H, et al. Multifactorial analysis of fertility after conservative laparoscopic treatment of ectopic pregnancy in a series of 223 patients. Fertil Steril 1991; 56:453.

Silva PD, Schaper AM, Rooney B. Reproductive outcome after 143 laparoscopic procedures for ectopic pregnancy. Obstet Gynecol 1993; 81:710.

Stovall TG, Ling FW, Carson SA, Buster JE. Serum progesterone and uterine curettage in differential diagnosis of ectopic pregnancy. *Fertil Steril*. Feb 1992;57(2):456-7.

S. N. Tripathy. The Fallopian Tubes. Jaypee Brothers Medical Pub; 1 edition. (July 2013).

Svare JA, Norup PA, Thomsen SG, Hornnes PJ, Maigaard S, Helm P, et al. [Heterotopic pregnancy after in vitro fertilization]. *Ugeskr Laeger*. Apr 11 1994;156(15):2230-3.

Van Den Eeden SK, Shan J, Bruce C, Glasser M. Ectopic pregnancy rate and treatment utilization in a large managed care organization. Obstet Gynecol 2005;105:1052–7.

Vermesh M, Silva PD, Rosen GF, et al. Management of unruptured ectopic gestation by linear salpingostomy: a prospective, randomized clinical trial of laparoscopy versus laparotomy. Obstet Gynecol 1989; 73:400.

Vinson DR. Emergency contraception and risk of ectopic pregnancy: is there need for extra vigilance?. *Ann Emerg Med*. Aug 2003;42(2):306-7.

Xu J, Kockanek KD, Murphy SL, et al. Deaths: final data for 2007. Natl Vital Stat Rep 2010;58:1–73. Available at www.cdc.gov/nchs/data/nvsr/nvsr58/nvsr58_19.pdf

Yao M, Tulandi T. Current status of surgical and nonsurgical management of ectopic pregnancy. Fertil Steril 1997; 67:421.

CPSIA information can be obtained at www.ICGtesting.com
Printed in the USA
LVOW05s1708300914

406587LV00008B/299/P